D0842769

Withdrawn

PINK RIBBON BLUES

PINK RIBBON BLUES

How Breast Cancer Culture Undermines Women's Health

GAYLE A. SULIK

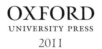

OXFORD
UNIVERSITY PRESS
2011

OXFORD
UNIVERSITY PRESS

Oxford University Press

Oxford University Press, Inc., publishes works that further
Oxford University's objective of excellence
in research, scholarship, and education.

Oxford New York
Auckland   Cape Town   Dar es Salaam   Hong Kong   Karachi
Kuala Lumpur   Madrid   Melbourne   Mexico City   Nairobi
New Delhi   Shanghai   Taipei   Toronto

With offices in
Argentina   Austria   Brazil   Chile   Czech Republic   France   Greece
Guatemala   Hungary   Italy   Japan Poland   Portugal   Singapore
South Korea   Switzerland   Thailand   Turkey   Ukraine   Vietnam

Published by Oxford University Press, Inc.
198 Madison Avenue, New York, New York 10016
www.oup.com

Library of Congress Cataloging-in-Publication Data
Sulik, Gayle A.
Pink ribbon blues: how breast cancer culture undermines women's health /
Gayle A. Sulik.
p. cm.
ISBN 978-0-19-974045-1
1. Breast–Cancer–Social aspects. 2. Health in mass media. 3. Women in mass
media. 4. Patient advocacy. I. Title.
RC280.B8S845 2011
362.196'99449—dc22
2010020255

Printed in the United States of America
on acid-free paper

10 9 8 7 6 5 4 3 2

For my Friend, Cathy Hoey

FOREWORD

"Pink culture" is ubiquitous. We are surrounded by pink ribbons that raise awareness about breast cancer and urge women to be screened against this deadly disease. In the marketplace, we are bombarded with "pink" products — pink sneakers, pink kitchen mixers, and even pink buckets of fried chicken — all designed to raise awareness and funds for breast cancer research and education. But is "pink culture" the best means to these ends? Are we doing the best we can to fight breast cancer?

Gayle Sulik's insightful book shows that optimistic claims about the decline in the breast cancer epidemic, the gains from new techniques of treatment and detection, and the promise of genomics and proteomics for personalized therapies mask insufficient data and moneyed interests while obscuring information about the causes of breast cancer. *Pink Ribbon Blues* provides an authoritative, evidence-based approach to distinguishing well-grounded hope from misleading hype. It examines the state of breast cancer advocacy today, and what it is – and is not – doing for women's health.

The grassroots breast cancer movement of twenty-plus years has been a force for progress for consumers interfacing with medicine. Over the years, much has changed in breast cancer biomedicine as well. Many of these changes have come from medical professionals and researchers who put the quality of life for women at the center of their concerns. The women's health movement that came to the public eye around 1970 with the publication of *Our Bodies, Ourselves,* for example, has played a crucial role in pushing the medical profession, government regulators, and researchers into treating women as active agents and potential experts of our own bodies. Much of the particular change in biomedicine came from obstreperous women, like Rose Kushner, insisting on being heard by their doctors and politicians, in the National Institutes of Health and in Congress.

By 1990, frustrated women raised their voices, opened their purses, and organized to get the attention of the public and of politicians in order to highlight shortfalls in progress against breast cancer. Despite reassurances from most quarters of the medical profession, women faced the harsh reality that mortality rates had not improved in 50 years. The breast cancer advocacy movement became a revolution to increase funding for innovative research; to question standard medical advice so that the public could learn about the complexities of the disease, including its known and suspected causes; to address the conditions of survivors' lives; and to dream of eliminating the disease for future generations.

We have much to learn from this extraordinary era and the many engaged citizens working to improve our health. Yet it is discouraging that, decades later, the same issues remain: Why are so many women living with, suffering from, and dying from breast cancer? What are the best ways to detect, treat, live with, and prevent this disease? Whose information is most reliable? What role, if any, should corporations play in disseminating medical information, encouraging particular modes of detection or treatment, or fund-raising for large breast cancer organizations? How do everyday messages about women and breast cancer survivorship help or diminish support for the diagnosed, or for those who are at risk? Whose voices are missing from the public debate? Where is the debate headed, and will it have any impact on the eradication of the disease?

Because we still cannot answer these challenging questions to our satisfaction, it is time to look at the problem with fresh insights. In order to increase our chances for improving quality of life, we must take stock of where we have been and where we are headed, re-evaluating the current culture and its powerful beliefs about what is best for women's health.

Gayle Sulik's thoughtful and provocative book gives us that opportunity. Her approach focuses us on the nexus of critical issues in women's and men's health, personal decision-making, and public policy. To understand the strengths and the limitations of the "pink ribbon culture" of breast cancer, Sulik looks at this complex cultural system it in its entirety, with its own language, norms, practices, and beliefs. She considers the history, the key players, the most prevalent messages, the key funders, and the most crucial outcomes of America's war on breast cancer. She listens to the words and stories of women who have breast cancer, the people who care about them, and those who are involved with breast cancer advocacy and education. She examines the advertising tableau and the imagery associated with pink culture. Then she carefully documents and analyzes the impact of this culture on the lives of women living with a breast cancer diagnosis. Finally, Sulik offers understanding about why pink ribbon culture has avoided public critique, and how society and advocacy together can regain crucial ground.

Gayle Sulik was a graduate student doing her master's degree in women's studies and her doctorate in sociology at the University at Albany, New York, when I first met her. She became a volunteer in the local breast cancer education and advocacy group I co-founded, the Capital Region Action Against Breast Cancer! (www.craab.org). Patricia Stocking Brown, another feminist biologist and the organizing force behind CRAAB!, committed us to a breast cancer agenda of strong scientific analysis as well as feminist values. Standing firmly in the legacy of the women's health movement, we wanted our organization to educate for better-informed decision-making. When we needed a new administrative director, Gayle was the obvious choice. She had been volunteering with the organization already, had solid research and organizational skills, was committed to understanding breast cancer holistically, and believed in compassionate care for the diagnosed. Gayle also was involved with creating the unique New York State Breast Cancer Network (www.nysbcsen.org). Through all of these efforts, Gayle honored the experiences and views of women with breast cancer, whether she agreed with them or not. Their voices became the foundation of her doctoral thesis and of this book.

As you weigh the evidence, consider the culture, and listen to the hundreds of survivors and fellow travelers Sulik interviewed over an eight-year period, *Pink Ribbon Blues* will help you to decide the best paths against breast cancer and related diseases. Sulik's methodology uses a qualitative approach, which allows patterns to emerge from data without super-imposing the researcher's beliefs, and her argument is grounded in primary, secondary, and historical data. She is fully aware that readers new to the constructive criticism of mainstream pink ribbon culture may find her analysis startling, even offensive. But keeping an open mind is essential to maintaining our foremost goal of eliminating breast cancer, and that is precisely what *Pink Ribbon Blues* beckons us to do.

Bonnie B. Spanier, Ph.D.,
Microbiology and Molecular Genetics
Emerita, Women's Studies Department,
University at Albany

ACKNOWLEDGEMENTS

This book has been almost ten years in the making. Though most of the writing of *Pink Ribbon Blues* took place in the last two years, my thinking about breast cancer and the pink ribbon began after I met Cathy Hoey and became a witness to her life and death with breast cancer. I hope she would be satisfied with the analysis presented in this book. It is dedicated to her, and to the many women who shared their experiences with me formally and informally as I tried to make sense of the growing and increasingly powerful pink ribbon culture. It is dedicated to those we have lost, and to those who continue to face breast cancer today — survivors, caregivers, friends, advocates, and those who search for new ways to treat and prevent this disease. There is no doubt that the desire to end breast cancer forever is a worthwhile and necessary goal. Lives are at stake. But the plausibility of reaching that goal has been diminished, not through a lack of effort, investment, visibility, or will but through misdirection and distraction. *Pink Ribbon Blues* is a call to refocus our attention to the people we seek to help, to the evidence we have amassed in the last thirty years, and to the strategies that would be most fruitful in achieving both our immediate and our ultimate aims.

This book was made possible with the support of the National Endowment for the Humanities. I received a 12-month research fellowship that allowed me to finalize my research and complete the manuscript. Any views, findings, conclusions, or recommendations expressed in *Pink Ribbon Blues* do not necessarily reflect those of the National Endowment for the Humanities. The analyses and arguments presented herein align with the endowment's goal of fostering greater understanding of the nation's culture through humanities projects of value to scholars and general audiences. I am grateful to the endowment for seeing the merit of this project and to Vassar College for encouraging me to apply.

I also received a research grant from Texas Woman's University to complete an in-depth analysis of breast cancer advertisements. I thank research assistant, Amber Deane, who searched, scanned, catalogued, and coded over three hundred full-page advertisements. Together, we clarified how breast cancer functioned in mass media as a brand name with a pink ribbon logo.

With deep gratitude, I thank the women and men who spoke freely and earnestly about their experiences with and opinions about breast cancer. The early data for this book came from a series of in-depth interviews starting in 2001 with sixty women in New York and Pennsylvania aged 31 to 79 who were diagnosed with different types and stages of breast cancer. These discussions were especially important for understanding how norms surrounding breast cancer influenced the decisions and everyday experiences of the diagnosed regardless of their level of involvement in pink ribbon culture, breast cancer advocacy, or social support programs. In the nine years that followed, I participated in an array of community awareness and fund-raising events, volunteered for a local breast cancer organization, attended educational panels oriented to different survivor and advocacy communities, worked with undergraduate students to explore health disparities and cultural competency in breast cancer information and resources, and attended local, regional, and national breast cancer conferences. Throughout this journey I spoke with hundreds of advocates, caregivers, health practitioners, researchers, and the diagnosed.

My advisors at the University at Albany (State University of New York) directed my dissertation on women's coping strategies and the care work involved in dealing with breast cancer. I thank Glenna Spitze, James Zetka, Ronald Jacobs, and Bonnie Spanier for their insightful critique and methodological guidance. Each of my advisors played an ongoing role as I developed peer-reviewed articles and presentations and expanded my ethnographic research to the broader pink ribbon culture. I especially want to thank Bonnie for reading every page of this manuscript to offer detailed comments. Her background as a microbiologist, women's health expert, breast cancer advocate, and feminist helped me to write about science in an accessible way, recount the history of breast cancer advocacy within the broader women's health movement, and write a balanced narrative that revealed the costs and benefits of how society has approached the breast cancer epidemic.

The anonymous reviewers of the scholarly journals *Qualitative Sociology, Gender & Society*, and *Sociology of Health and Illness* and their editors Javier Auyero, Dana Britton, and Clive Seale offered comments that informed and contextualized my analyses on care, coping, biomedicine, and identity that were later foundational for this book. Susan Chambre and Melinda Goldner gave valuable feedback on the cultural and institutional transformations in health care for a new edited volume (10) of *Advances in Medical Sociology*. Astrid Eich-Krohm, co-author and friend, challenged my thinking beyond breast cancer to consider how health information about a variety of women's health issues may empower but also pressure women into using health services that may not improve the quality of their lives.

I am thankful to the friends and colleagues who offered insight and critique of the various ideas that culminated in this book: Osama Abi-Mershed, Judy Adkison, Kristina Balabuch, Monica Batkis-O'Donnell, Brian Beck, Chris Bobel, Ann Boodt, Kim Booker, Christine Bose, Sunita Bose, Patricia Stocking

Brown, Phil Brown, Starr Campbell, Capital Region Action Against Breast Cancer, Kathy Charmaz, Esther Chow, Adele Clarke, Jeannine Coffey, Denise Copelton, Leslie Dunn, Leslie Enlow, Susan Ferguson, Donna Gardner, Janet Gray, Diane Harriford, Joseph Hefta, Barbara Hokamp, Carla Howery, Michael Hutton, DiAnna Hynds, Dionne Jackson, Barbara Katz Rothman, Theresa Kendall, Jessica Kenty-Drane, Minjeong Kim, Becky Klett, Pamela Lehman, Clarence Lu, Kate Linnenberg, Anna Love, Candice Lowe, Gale Miller, Hannah MacIntyre, Sarah MacIntyre, Marque Miringoff, Omar Nagy, Margaret Nelson, Misti Patton, Barbara Ray, Margaret Roberts, Christie Roden, Linda Rubin, Maureen Saringer, Phyllis Minton, Joan Sheehan, William Smith, Jan Spence, Marybeth Stalp, Jennifer Tirrell, Beverly Yuen Thompson, Lee Anne Todd, Barry Trachtenberg, Beth Tracton-Bishop, Margaret Vitullo, Matthew Wheeler, Susann Wheeler, Rebecca Williams, Audra Wolfe, Rebecca Woodland, and Philip Yang.

My editor at Oxford University Press, Regan Hoffman, inspired me from the beginning of our relationship together. I knew she understood what the book was about when she remarked that after reading the proposal she had "one of those rare moments of realization where you can't quite believe you'd never considered things in that way before." Aha moments are life changing, and I hope every reader of *Pink Ribbon Blues* reaches this kind of clarity. I thank Regan and the entire team at OUP who enthusiastically and skillfully worked on the production of this book.

I owe a large debt to my family who supported this work over the last decade and accepted that I would be tied to my desk for hours, days, and weeks at a time. To my mother Gail, my father Pete, my grandmothers Doris, Margaret, and Vinnie, my grandfathers Charles, Peter, and Elmer, my sister Allison, my parents-in-law Carmen and Julian, my step-father Richard, and my extended family who, with too many people to list, were happy to know that Gayle Ann found her calling as a writer. Thank you all.

I leave my final statement of gratitude for my husband, Julian. It is fitting that I write this on our anniversary for it was his encouragement, steadfastness, support, and love that allowed me to find my voice as a writer, live my vision as a researcher, and trust in the process of unfolding that is the foundation for any worthwhile piece of writing. Julian has read almost every word I have ever written. He is my beloved and my muse.

CONTENTS

Pink Ribbon Blues

ONE

WHAT IS PINK RIBBON CULTURE?

*Almost all of the eye-level space has been filled with photocopied
bits of cuteness and sentimentality: pink ribbons, a cartoon about
a woman with iatrogenically flattened breasts, an "Ode to a
Mammogram," a list of the "Top Ten Things Only Women
Understand" ("Fat Clothes" and "Eyelash Curlers" among them),
and, inescapably, right next to the door, the poem "I Said a Prayer
for You Today," illustrated with pink roses.*

BARBARA EHRENREICH, WELCOME TO CANCERLAND

Having been diagnosed with breast cancer, journalist
Barbara Ehrenreich wrote a thought-provoking article
for *Harper's Magazine* in 2001 that described her personal introduction to the world of breast cancer.[1] The culture that
Ehrenreich described as she waited in a changing room to have
a mammogram was far more complex and omnipresent than
I had realized: the ultra-feminine pink kitsch of the breast cancer
marketplace, the infantilizing trope of teddy bears and tote
bags, the mainstreaming of support as united sentimentality,
the battle cry of survivorship coupled with the tyranny of cheerfulness, disease and its treatment as a rite of passage and chance

for creative self-transformation, the promise of medical technology, the cancer–industrial complex, and the denigration of death and the dying. This vivid account described a new American religion just for women, replete with traditionally feminine symbolism, ritual, and doctrine.

Ehrenreich's critical observation of breast cancer sparked a public discussion of the corporate interest in breast cancer, the dilution of feminist ideals within the breast cancer movement, the feminine aesthetic of mainstream breast cancer culture, and mass obedience to medical protocols. Although the discussion provoked outrage, concern, and critical evaluation on the part of some, a culture of breast cancer survivorship continued to gain social, economic, and political force.

The pink ribbon culture that exists today is a unique cultural system. With roots in the women's health movement of the 1970s and the breast cancer movement of the 1980s and 1990s, pink ribbon culture flourishes as a new dimension of American culture with its own symbols, beliefs, values, norms, and practices. Support groups, educational programs, community events, and breast cancer–related services convey elements of pink ribbon culture. At the same time, breast cancer holds a prominent position in mass media, the cancer industry, and corporate cause-marketing. Pink ribbon paraphernalia saturate shopping malls, billboards, magazines, television, and other entertainment venues. Having gone mainstream, pink ribbon culture is now widely available to a virtual community of breast cancer survivors, would-be supporters, and the general public. The identity of the warrior who fights courageously against breast cancer is open to anyone who buys, displays, or thinks pink.

Prior to 2001, my knowledge about breast cancer was slight. When I was in high school in the 1980s, the 28-year-old sister of one of my friends had been diagnosed with breast cancer, and she died about a year later. I didn't know much of what went on, and I didn't ask. It was just a strange, quiet mystery. After I went to college, my childhood piano teacher, who had been a weekly part of my life for about 8 years as I stumbled around the keyboard until I could one day play Chopin's *Fantasy in C Sharp Minor*, was diagnosed with breast cancer. When I went to see her on my break, she had already been in treatment for several months. I remembered her as a kind-hearted taskmaster. We never talked much about anything besides the music, but I felt close to her. When I saw her laying on a cot in the front room of her house, barely able to move, with a thin face and a bandana on her head, I didn't know what to say, how to feel, or how to respond. In all those years, I had never even been in that room. There was no piano. There was no music. She died several weeks after my visit.

A full 10 years went by before I thought about breast cancer again. One of my coworkers was diagnosed with breast cancer when she was 30, and she had a recurrence 5 years later. I met her just after she started treatment again, and we quickly became coffee buddies. We never met for other social occasions or invited anyone to join us. We simply met, and had very long conversations while drinking coffee. We covered a wide range of

subjects from great recipes, to difficulties at work, to philosophies about marriage and family, to the places we'd love to visit,
to what inspired us, to our purpose in life. Sometimes I would
ask her about her chemotherapy treatments. And sometimes, she
wouldn't just change the subject away from what I knew was a
constant and arduous experience for her. Cathy generally kept
her diagnosis and treatment quiet, and she was not involved in
support groups or advocacy organizations. When I found out
about a community-based organization nearby, I thought it
might be a good way for me to learn more about breast cancer,
so that I could be a better support for my friend. Cathy was
always interested to hear what I had learned.

When Cathy's treatments became more intensive, she stopped
working and spent most of her time at home. Instead of meeting at the café, we would have our coffee conversations at her
house, often without the coffee. We'd sit at the kitchen table and
talk for hours. Her dog, Scooter, would usually sit at her feet
and then do a little dance for the promise of a snack. He adored
Cathy, and his antics always put a smile on both of our faces.
At one point Cathy started giving me things…a cookbook, a
vase, things from her kitchen. It hadn't occurred to me at the
time that she was giving her things away because she knew her
time was limited. She talked more frequently about her treatments, the mistakes she had made in her life, and how most
people had no idea what it was like to have cancer. She would
get very animated when I talked about my plans, my commitments, my beloved, and my hopes for the future. It was as if we

were both transported from her little kitchen to some grand and important adventure.

A few weeks after her 40th birthday, just around Thanksgiving, Cathy's doctors told her that there was nothing more they could do. The cancer was growing out of control despite the toxic chemical therapies she had been given, so they finally stopped her treatment. Within 6 weeks she died. The last day I saw Cathy was just a few days before her death. She hadn't been out of bed in weeks, but as soon as she saw me she tried to get up. She wanted to make me some tea. As she tried to get out of bed, I insisted that I had been sufficiently caffeinated and tried not to cry. I apologized as my eyes welled up. She said, "It's okay." My dying friend was trying to comfort me. This only made me cry more. Unlike our usual meetings, this one did not include much conversation. I just sat at her bedside as Cathy dozed in and out, and we shared the quiet weight of her reality. I told her I would visit her again in a few days, and she smiled. She died before I had the chance. After the funeral I went to her house. Scooter had stolen the hat Cathy had been wearing for past 6 weeks to keep warm. He kept it under his chin and wouldn't let anyone near it. I think he knew she wasn't coming back and was just as sad we were.

When Cathy died, I was consumed with grief. One evening I went to a business meeting at the breast cancer organization where I had been volunteering and noticed that I could barely keep my attention on the conversation. After the meeting I walked out with Pat Brown who was on the board of directors, one of the founders of the organization, and a breast cancer survivor. When I told her about my friend's death and my difficulty concentrating, she said in a matter-of-fact yet thoughtful manner that she had envisioned her own death. She wrote a eulogy, imagined her funeral, and tried to come to terms with the fact that she was going to die—and that most likely she would die from breast cancer. She said, "After I faced my death in my own mind, I could get on with the work I had to do. Your friend probably faced her death long before she died." From that brief conversation, I reached new understanding.

How we face death says a lot about how we live our lives, and fear of death can impede action as well as shape it. Now I see that Cathy, along with my piano teacher and my friend's sister, had a significant influence on my own consciousness about breast cancer. My memories of them, along with the experiences I've had with the hundreds of people I know who are living with or who have died from breast cancer, inform and ground my social analysis. Sociologist John Lofland and his colleagues call this process "starting where you are." In making "problematic" in our research that which is problematic in our lives, researchers' personal experiences can contribute to their understanding of the comparable experiences of those studied.[2] Making sense of pink ribbon culture in a way that bears upon my own experiences and those of people I care about helps me to understand better the relevance of American society's war on breast cancer.

Pink ribbon culture is problematic. This book explains why.

Pink Ribbon Blues looks within and beneath pink ribbon culture to examine how it works, what it creates, and how it affects the experience of breast cancer for survivors and supporters. Pink ribbon culture in the United States has become more than a cultural trend or a successful industry: it has become a distinct cultural system that is integrated into the fabric of American life. Grounded in advocacy, deeply held beliefs about gender and femininity, mass-mediated consumption, and the cancer industry, pink ribbon culture has transformed breast cancer from an important social problem that requires complicated social and medical solutions to a popular item for public consumption. Beyond its representation of breast cancer awareness, the pink ribbon has become an iconic symbol with the ideological power to turn breast cancer into a brand name with a recognizable logo. Although breast cancer advocacy has moved breast cancer into the light and empowered millions of women to claim their status as survivors, pink ribbon culture inadvertently helps to maintain a war on breast cancer that has little chance of ending in the near future. The goal to eradicate breast cancer simply is not being realized.

The chief executive of the American Cancer Society, John R. Seffrin, balks at the conclusion that little progress has been made in the war on cancer. In response to an article published on April 24, 2009 in *The New York Times*, which called "advances" in the 40-year war on cancer "elusive," Seffrin immediately wrote a letter to the editor refuting the statement. He wrote: "The progress we're making against cancer is unmistakable. Cancer death rates have dropped 18 percent among men and 10 percent among women since 1990-91. During that time, more than half a million deaths were avoided."[3] Similarly, the National Cancer Institute reports that 55 to 66 percent of all cancer patients today can expect to live for 5 or more years after the diagnosis, up from about 50 percent in 1979.[4] Clearly, there has been overall progress since President Nixon officially declared the war on cancer. However, these improvements have not been equally distributed across different types of cancers at all stages of disease.

Medical advancements, diagnostic screening, and preventive practices have been responsible for reductions in mortality and/or incidence rates for childhood cancers, colorectal cancer, and lung cancer. Mortality rates for childhood cancers have declined by almost 50 percent since 1975, and more children are living longer after diagnosis.[5] The American Cancer Society attributes the substantial progress in pediatric cancer survival rates to improved treatments and a high proportion of patient participation in clinical trials. For colorectal cancer, mortality rates have declined in both men and women over the past two decades by 1.8 percent per year from 1985 to 2002, and 4.7 percent per year from 2002 to 2004. This decrease reflects declining incidence rates and improvements in early detection and treatment.[6] Although the number of deaths from lung cancer increased from 156,900 in 2000 to 161,840 in 2008, death rates among men decreased by 1.3 percent per year from 1990 to 1994, and by 2.0 percent per year from 1994 to 2004. After continuously increasing for several decades, death rates among women are now beginning to stabilize.[7] More than anything else, trends in lung cancer mortality reflect a general decrease in smoking over the past 30 years.

Although medical advancements, screening, and prevention efforts have improved health outcomes for some cancers, this is not the case for breast cancer. There was a 40 percent increase in diagnoses and a near doubling of early-stage breast cancers from 1973 to 1998, corresponding to a rise in mammography screening.[8] Death rates declined by 2.5 percent annually for white women between 1994 and 2003 and 1.4 percent for African American women.[9] Since 1990, there have been larger decreases in death rates for women younger than age 50 (3.3 percent per year) compared to women age 50 and older (2.0 percent per year). According to the *American Cancer Society Facts and Figures* for 2008, the decrease in breast cancer death rates "represents progress in both earlier detection and improved treatment."[10] Yet the increase in early-stage diagnoses does not translate to a corresponding decline in late-stage cancers, as would be expected if early detection were successful in preventing the development of more advanced (and less curable) cancers later on. In addition, the 5-year survival for stage zero cancers, which are not life-threatening, is 100 percent, making survival statistics look better than they are. Every year over 40,000 women and 450 men die from breast cancer.[11]

Knowing that this may be difficult to consider, I suggest that several aspects of the mainstream pink ribbon culture have impeded progress in the war on breast cancer:

- Scientific controversies that could inform medical practices and research agendas tend to be avoided or simplified for the eyes of the public, particularly the survival benefits of mammography, the multifaceted causes, and the reality that there are no guaranteed modes of prevention or treatment.
- Profit motives largely define pink ribbon culture within the context of a multi-billion-dollar cancer industry, which itself has many profit centers, including the pharmaceutical industry, the medical system, technology manufacturers, large breast cancer organizations, and sponsoring corporations.
- The widely distributed imagery of millions of participants, who walk or run for a cure every year donning smiling faces and pink paraphernalia, does not reflect the illness experience of the millions of diagnosed women who do not fit neatly into the pink breast cancer box.

As breast cancer advocacy was repackaged for mass distribution through a widely disseminated pink ribbon culture, these and other consequences largely fell beneath the radar.

The good news is that all of the public attention to breast cancer has raised a substantial amount of money for research and support programs, and mobilized millions of survivors and supporters to take action. Where we spend our research dollars, how we define support, and the kinds of actions we take next will go a long way toward determining whether the war on breast cancer will have any chance of ending in the 21st century. There are several factors that must be acknowledged and dealt with if pink ribbon culture is to fulfill its promise of eradicating breast cancer forever while supporting diagnosed women in the meantime.

First, we must acknowledge that the breast cancer movement is not a unitary, consensual force represented by a singular organization. There are hundreds if not thousands of community-based groups and organizations across the nation mobilizing to provide support services, fill gaps in care, help diagnosed people to understand complex medical information, seek precautionary measures, inform the public about cancer, and advocate for specific public policies aimed at improving the quality of care and opening the access points in the healthcare system. Some of these organizations are committed to changing the system itself. Fueled by their membership, volunteer work, grant funding, pro bono work, local fundraisers, and sometimes corporate sponsorship, these organizations are the grassroots of the breast cancer movement. Their missions and agendas are sometimes in alignment with the mammoth organizations visible in pink ribbon culture, but often they are not. For pink ribbon culture to represent the breast cancer movement, it must be reflexive and responsive to the needs of all kinds of breast cancer survivors and supporters who are caring for their communities and organizing for social change.

We must also listen to the voices that are routinely omitted or marginalized from pink ribbon culture. Voices can be heard through organizations, but they are also present in the personal stories (illness narratives) of breast cancer survivors. The stories people tell and write about their illnesses give a function to the illness that helps them to make sense of its effects on their lives and futures. Some stories are revered in pink ribbon culture. Those that focus on overcoming adversity and being a better person because of it can be found in numerous survivor profiles, biographies, poems, and other cultural representations that circulate in the pink mainstream. Sober accounts that reveal realism, cynicism, ongoing struggle, or death often fall on the margins. These kinds of stories can be hard to tell and hard to hear, but these are the stories that authenticate the diversity of illness experiences and open the potential for new ways of thinking about breast cancer, new ways of coping, and new ways of providing support.

Second, we must recognize the role gender plays in pink ribbon culture. What does it mean to mark breast cancer with the color pink? The color pink signifies the innocence and sometimes childishness, nurturance, emotional sensitivity, and selflessness associated with traditional femininity. It also symbolizes the feminine half of heterosexuality and a love of feminine accoutrements. Inscribing breast cancer survivorship, support, and awareness activities with pink femininity draws upon and reactivates societal gender expectations. For example, images abound of a sisterhood of courageous women draped in pink, enthusiastically supporting one another, selflessly organized, and optimistically calling attention to the need for awareness, research, and funding in the battle against breast cancer. Gender expectations about women's innate selflessness encourage them to put the needs of others first, even when they are sick or diagnosed with cancer. In reality, selflessness pressures diagnosed women to engage in a "balancing act" as they continually assess when, and under what conditions, they should put others second and instead think about themselves.

Pink also references a society that celebrates women's breasts as the principal symbol of womanhood, motherhood, and female sexuality. Since breast cancer places the social integrity of a woman's body in jeopardy, restoring the feminine body (or at least normalizing its appearance) is a sign of victory in the war on breast cancer. Wigs, makeup, fashion, prosthetic breasts, and reconstruction help women to maintain a socially accept-able feminine appearance. This norm forces women to choose between devaluing their bodies (I don't need my breasts anymore anyway), hyper-valuing their bodies (Without breasts I don't feel like a whole woman), or viewing their scars as a badge of honor. The dominant representations in pink ribbon culture reinforce these messages within the auspices of broader gender expectations that value younger women's healthy bodies for their sexual primacy and devalue older women's bodies or disabled women's bodies because they are thought to be devoid of sexual usefulness. Thinking of scars, or an otherwise disfig-ured body, as a symbol of struggle or victory (but not beauty) is the only culturally justified way to accept women's bodily disorder.

Not all women want to (or are able to) conform to the three options above. Pink ribbon culture solves this problem by integrating the masculine and the feminine. The masculine ethos in American cancer culture uses the war metaphor to emphasize a model of survivorship steeped in the masculine-identified qualities of strength, courage, and aggressiveness. In contrast, the feminine ethos resists the war metaphor in favor of nurturance, empathy, and a relational orientation. Uniting these competing standpoints, pink ribbon culture has created a unique model of breast cancer survivorship in the form of the "she-ro." With femininity intact, either through normalization processes or using breast cancer as a badge of honor, the she-ro is a feminine hero with the attitude, style, and verve to kick cancer's butt while wearing 6-inch heels and pink lipstick. She returns from the battle, if not victorious, then revitalized and transcendent. Most of the diagnosed women I have met do not fit this description, but some of them aspire to it.

The prevalence of she-roic models in pink ribbon culture contributes to a general lack of understanding about what it means to hear the words, "you have breast cancer." It creates the impression that diagnosed women should feel proud of their experience and use it for transformative purposes. Pride and transformation require optimism, the cornerstone of survivorship. Sociologist Arlie Hochschild writes about the "feeling rules" that govern how people try to feel or try *not* to feel in a given situation (such as feeling happy at weddings and sad at funerals).[12] In pink ribbon culture, feeling rules govern how best to fight the war on breast cancer. Optimism translates to a brand of social support that almost demands commodification of the illness and a model of survivorship focused on acquiescence to mainstream ideals.

Barbara Ehrenreich refers to the mandate to be cheerful as a form of tyranny that can take women unawares when facing what is cast as, and what may be, mortal danger. For the 77 percent of women who are diagnosed with invasive breast cancer—defined as such because of its capacity to spread—it can be very discouraging to be "bright-sided."[13] I empathize when the first thing I see upon entering a grocery store is a cascade of pink ribbon balloons hanging from the ceiling, pink shopping bags, and a table full of sugary baked goods slathered in hot pink frosting. Is breast cancer really so festive?

Not according to an article in the *Boston Globe Sunday Magazine*. With the title "Sick of Pink," the article tells the stories of several diagnosed women who are not enamored with the sea of pink ribbons and products that invade public spaces, especially during National Breast Cancer Awareness Month. One woman, diagnosed at age 24, described her self-imposed pop-culture blackout during the month of October when she tries to avoid TV, magazines, and especially shopping. She said, "I want to buy my English muffins and not be reminded of [my cancer]… I felt kind of hateful."[14] While many people wrote in support of the article's message that perhaps some companies were using women's pain to increase profits, one response in particular revealed the anger and defensiveness that can occur when anyone, including the diagnosed, raises questions about whether the ends (alleged research dollars) justify the means (cause-marketing and pink ribbon culture):

> I really find it incredible that people are actually complaining about receiving donations from corporations. Breast Cancer generates more awareness and charitable donations than ANY other fatal disease in the US. They keep talking about being disrespected or used… HOW ABOUT BEING GRATEFUL PEOPLE CARE ENOUGH TO BUY THOSE ANNOYING PINK PRODUCTS!!

The response by "eoleary29" is a harsh and thoughtless rebuke of the breast cancer survivors who went against the grain of optimism to reveal their feelings of distress and concern.

Pink ribbon culture is geared more toward encouraging people to feel good about the cause than to acknowledge the often difficult and un-pretty realities of breast cancer diagnosis and treatment. In this type of cultural environment, the diagnosed must carefully decide what to reveal about their illness experiences, and what to hide. Questioning the pink status quo, as the article did, seems to call into question the good intentions and symbolic gestures of those who consciously buy and display pink. Pink ribbon culture reinforces this kind of either/or thinking. Either pink ribbon culture and the people who participate in it are all good, or they must be all bad. Instead, I suggest we must claim a middle ground. Pink ribbon culture is like any other cultural system. It has both intended and unintended consequences. If both are identified, then people can determine how to maximize the benefits and minimize the costs.

This brings me to the third point. For pink ribbon culture to fulfill its promise, we must consider the role of the cancer industry on pink ribbon culture and the financial incentives that keep the war on breast cancer profitable. It is no coincidence that the American Cancer Society's National Breast Cancer Awareness Month (NBCAM), which first promoted mammography screening, was sponsored by the subsidiary of one of the world's largest multinational chemical corporations. Zeneca Group plc, of Imperial Chemical Industries, later merged with pharmaceutical giant Astra AB to become one of the wealthiest members of the breast cancer industry through the development and sale of oncology drugs. Still the sponsor of NBCAM, along with the American Cancer Society, the conflict of interest between sponsoring breast cancer awareness programs while profiting from breast cancer diagnosis and treatment and/or contributing to a carcinogenic environment is one of the many competing interests that undermine pink ribbon culture.

The American Cancer Society publicly stated in an article in *The New York Times* (October 21, 2009) that the benefits of detecting many cancers, especially breast cancer and prostate cancer, have been overstated. Chief medical officer of the American Cancer Society Dr. Otis Brawley said: "I'm admitting that American medicine has overpromised when it comes to screening.

The advantages to screening have been exaggerated."[15] For every 2,000 women screened in a 10-year period, ten women will be treated unnecessarily and only one woman will have her life prolonged.[16] Brawley's acknowledgment of scientific evidence that has been the center of a heated scientific discussion since 2000-2001 is a major shift from the American Cancer Society's long-term commitment to screening. It remains to be seen whether the American Cancer Society and other staunch supporters of mammography screening will revise their screening recommendations in accord with this acknowledgment. The message that mammography screening leads to early detection and "early detection saves lives" has been the touchstone of the most highly visible breast cancer awareness activities since the mid-1980s.

Habits are hard to break, especially when they are institutionalized. Within just 7 days of the American Cancer Society's unprecedented statement, I received the following automated message on my cell phone from my insurance provider, Blue Cross Blue Shield of Texas:

> One in eight women will be diagnosed with breast cancer in her lifetime. Most doctors agree that early detection tests for breast cancer save many thousands of lives each year. If you have not had a mammogram in the past year, we encourage you to contact your network primary care doctor or OBGYN and schedule this important screening. In addition to a mammogram every one to two years, yearly breast exams by your doctor are important for the early detection of breast cancer.

> Remember: Early detection can result in the successful treatment of breast cancer.

Since mammography screening has become a central organizing principle of the war on breast cancer in pink ribbon culture, it is very difficult to suggest that it may not be the answer. Asking what is at stake, and for whom, will help us to unravel the uses and misuses of medical technologies, practices, and protocols.

The use of breast cancer in cause-marketing similarly produces conflicts of interest between breast cancer advocacy and corporate sponsorships outside of the medical system. Samantha King's exposé in *Pink Ribbons, Inc.* reveals the thriving relationship between nonprofit breast cancer organizations and corporate partners, a trend that has grown substantially even in the past 5 years. The programs and strategies that dominate pink ribbon culture stress philanthropy and civic participation while capitalizing on American generosity in the name of the breast cancer cause.[17] King argues that strategic corporate philanthropy has benefited corporations while co-opting the breast cancer movement, promoting a celebratory discourse of survivorship, shifting attention away from prevention and environmental causes, and masking the decline of public funding for social services and research support.

While cause-marketing has further increased attention to the cause, raised funds for some prominent organizations and medical research projects, pleased many conscientious consumers, and benefited major corporations and almost any individual or group that posts a pink ribbon, it has also contributed to the obfuscation of the diversity of the breast cancer movement, the femininization of the illness, and the profitability of breast cancer for the cancer industry and other corporate interests—the first three factors undermining the potential of pink ribbon culture to achieve its primary goal.

None of this would be possible to this extent without mass media. The cause of breast cancer has garnered extensive media attention in a wide range of outlets, including news, entertainment, and advertising. Much of pink ribbon culture is now transmitted through an array of marketing strategies and modes of consumption that rely heavily on mass media to influence potential audiences and consumers. In fact, breast cancer is an illness that now functions as a concept brand. Different from most brands, such as Nike or Coke, the *breast cancer brand* does not involve a single company or product line; instead, it draws from a collection of symbols, images, and meanings within pink ribbon culture to maintain the principal message that breast cancer is a vitally important cause, and that supporting it indicates good will toward women. The brand encourages people to buy and display pink in the name of increased awareness, improvement in women's lives, faith in medical science, and hope for a future without breast cancer.

The first part of this book shows how pink ribbon culture provides the cultural platform and discursive framework through which gender, mass media, and consumption operate to fuel the breast cancer industry. Media saturation and pink consumption have enabled pink ribbon culture to saturate American society, further contributing to its normalization and invisibility. Idealized portrayals of breast cancer survivors and their supporters strengthen these pillars and guide public perceptions. The result is a narrow set of expectations, values, and ideas about the meaning of breast cancer awareness, support, and survivorship. This section offers a critique of the pink ribbon culture, identifying the underlying assumptions, processes, and consequences that enable pink ribbon culture to preserve its status and power in shaping how individuals, the public, mass media, the medical system, government agencies, and the cancer industry understand and approach breast cancer.

The second part of the book draws together key themes and highlights an emerging tension within pink ribbon culture as the context of breast cancer in the United States continues to shift. For two decades, the epic story of the she-ro has functioned as a canon within illness narratives. Pink ribbon culture aggressively markets the she-ro's "common experience" and her cultural and scientific toolbox for dealing with the disease. This approach has not succeeded in preventing or eradicating breast cancer, providing access to quality treatment and care, offering adequate and inclusive support or representation for the diagnosed, or managing conflicts of interest between advocacy, care, and profit. Thus, the she-ro is no longer contextually relevant for increasing numbers of people. Although key organizations and institutions in pink ribbon culture are striving to maintain dominance through the proliferation of norms and messages that discourage public scrutiny, a growing number of individuals and groups are striving to create and model change in the status quo.

This book is based upon 8 years of ethnographic observation, analysis of breast cancer advertisements and awareness campaigns, and interviews with hundreds of breast cancer survivors, supporters, advocates, and caregivers. What the reader will find in the following pages are detailed observations and descriptions of the pink ribbon culture, historical perspectives, examples of cultural artifacts and media messages, pertinent medical information and scientific controversies, financial data, and excerpts that reveal deeply felt and open conversations with those who are part of this culture and those who are not.

NOTES

1. B. Ehrenreich, "Welcome to Cancerland," *Harper's Magazine* (2001).

2. J. Lofland, D. Snow, L. Anderson, & L. Lofland, *Analyzing Social Settings: A Guide to Qualitative Observation and Analysis* (Thomson Wadsorth, 2006, 4th ed.), 10.

3. Editorial Desk, "Fighting Cancer: Who's Winning?" *The New York Times*, April 29, 2009.

4. National Cancer Institute, U.S. National Institutes of Health, "Surveillance Epidemiology and End Results (SEER): SEER Stat Fact Sheets." www.cancer.gov; M. J. Horner, L. A. G. Ries, M. Krapcho,

N. Neyman, R. Aminou, N. Howlader, S. F. Altekruse, E. J. Feuer, L. Huang, A. Mariotto, B. A. Miller, D. R. Lewis, M. P. Eisner, D. G. Stinchcomb, & B. K. Edwards (Eds.), *SEER Cancer Statistics Review*, 1975-2006, National Cancer Institute. Bethesda, MD. http://seer.cancer. gov/csr/1975_2006/, based on November 2008 SEER data submission, posted to the SEER web site, 2009. The overall 5-year relative survival rate for 1999 to 2005 determined from 17 SEER geographic areas.

5. Cancer Incidence and Survival Among Children and Adolescents: United States SEER Program 1975-1995 http://seer.cancer.gov/publications/childhood/; *American Cancer Society. Cancer Facts and Figures:* 2008.

6. Ibid.

7. American Cancer Society. Cancer Facts and Figures: 2008 and Cancer Facts and Figures: 2000.

8. E. J. Feuer & L. Wun, "How Much of the Recent Rise in Breast Cancer Incidence Can Be Explained by Increases in Mammography Utilization? A Dynamic Population Model Approach," *American Journal of Epidemiology*, 136, no. 12 (1992): 1423-36.

9. L. A. G. Ries, M. P. Eisner, & C. L. Kosary (Eds.), *SEER Fast Stats: Breast Cancer* 1994-2003. National Cancer Institute. Bethesda, MD (2006).

10. American Cancer Society, *Cancer Facts and Figures* 2008. Atlanta, GA (2008), 9.

11. American Cancer Society. *Cancer Facts and Figures* 2008. Atlanta, GA (2008).

12. A. Hochschild, *The Managed Heart: The Commercialization of Human Feeling* (University of California Press, 2003).

13. B. Ehrenreich, Bright-sided: How the Relentless Promotion of Positive Thinking Has Undermined America (Macmillan, 2009).

14. K. *Frieswick*, "Sick of Pink," *The Boston Globe Sunday Magazine*, October 3, 2009. http://www.boston.com/bostonglobe/magazine/articles/2009/10/04/sick_of_pink/

15. G. Kolata, "Cancer Society, in Shift, Has Concerns on Screenings." *The New York Times*, October 21, 2009. http://www.nytimes.com/2009/10/21/health/21cancer.html?_r=2&em.

16. P. C. Gotzsche & M. Nielsen, "Screening for Breast Cancer with Mammography," *Cochrane Database of Systematic Reviews*, 4 (2006). http://www.cochrane.org/reviews/en/ab001877.html.

17. J. Fosket, A. Karran, & C. LaFia, "Breast Cancer in Popular Women's Magazines from 1913-1996," in *Breast Cancer: Society Shapes an Epidemic*, ed. S. Ferguson and A. Kasper, 303-324. (New York: St. Martin's Press, 2000); S. King, *Pink Ribbons, Inc.: Breast Cancer and the Politics of Philanthropy* (Minneapolis: University of Minnesota Press, 2006); M. Klawiter, "Breast Cancer in Two Regimes: The Impact of Social Movements on Illness Experience," *Sociology of Health & Illness* 26 (September) (2004): 845-74.

TWO

THE DEVELOPMENT OF PINK RIBBON CULTURE

Denial of [breast cancer] had been ingrained in the culture for so long that resistance to it had become second nature. Any woman drawing attention to her own cancer brought disgrace not just on herself but on everyone else with the disease...Shame itself proved to be contagious. Given these obstacles, the surprise may not be that it took so long for women to speak out but rather that they ever had the courage to do it at all.

ELLEN LEOPOLD, A DARKER RIBBON[1]

The public character of breast cancer in today's culture provides sharp relief to the stigma that was associated with the disease prior to the 1970s.[2] For decades, breast cancer had been a negatively characterized condition that conferred deviant status to diagnosed women. In addition to high mortality and a corresponding fear that breast cancer was synonymous with a death sentence, the taboo surrounding breast cancer intensified medical and social mores that promoted women's dependence on paternalistic medicine. Authoritative doctor–patient relationships, inaccessible medical language, invasive procedures, lack of concern for women patients, and the predominance of male models of disease heightened medical control over breast cancer and the women who were diagnosed.[3] Social norms associated with the feminine mystique further supported proper etiquette and dress that promoted women's compliance and masked the presence of the disease.[4] Socially isolated, most diagnosed women were unaware of other women with breast cancer. Open discussion of breast cancer, networks of social support, access to information, and empowered decision-making would have been unimaginable.

THE BREAST CANCER MOVEMENT

For breast cancer to move out of the private sphere and into the public, the stigma had to be removed. The women's, patients', and consumers' rights movements of the 1970s encouraged patient empowerment, the development of lay medical knowledge, and a commitment to sharing information with other women. They also began to question medical authority, demand information about medical procedures, and insist on patients' rights in medical decision-making.[5] Increased discussion and local organizing fueled the expansion of assistance programs and organizations. As organizing began to take a more political tone, breast cancer survivors formalized their networks to influence policy and medical practice, and to institutionalize funding streams and support systems. What transpired was a vibrant and successful social movement, and diagnosed women were at the center of it.

By the early 1990s, the breast cancer movement claimed a more public character. In addition to increased media attention, advocacy groups were involved with research programs and support services, and the advancement of legislative issues related to federal funding, quality breast cancer care, and patients' rights. Working to ensure that attention to breast cancer was not fleeting, the new National Breast Cancer Coalition (NBCC) advanced legislation to establish the Department of Defense Peer-Reviewed Breast Cancer Research Program in 1993, and was largely responsible for the program's annual funding increases to date. Totaling $2.1 billion since its inception, this program involves the active participation of breast cancer survivors in reviewing proposals for breast cancer research. Claiming a seat at the table has made certain that diagnosed women could on some level have greater influence on the medical practices and research agendas that affected them.

The breast cancer movement was committed to de-stigmatizing the disease, increasing awareness, promoting informed decision-making, distributing accurate and accessible information, providing emotional and practical support, challenging medical authority, and exposing medical practices to public scrutiny. Once breast cancer was out in the open, however, the trajectory started to shift. The increased presence and visibility of resources and support groups, changes in public policy, and heightened media exposure elevated breast cancer's social status from disease to epidemic. With this high level of social importance, the movement had more clout, as did the identity of the breast cancer survivor. Local organizing and group dynamics started to become incorporated into an overarching "culture of survivorship" oriented to optimism, personal empowerment, and the "survivor" as an identity category.[6] As the culture of survivorship was repackaged for mass distribution, the principles, strategies, and accomplishments of the breast cancer movement developed into a broader pink ribbon culture. Despite ongoing resistance from within the movement, mass dissemination diluted and homogenized breast cancer advocacy and the culture it produced. Key organizations and their missions became institutionalized into the broader cancer establishment.[7]

Merging advocacy and industry, the resultant pink ribbon culture has become a dynamic and highly public dimension of American culture that relies on mass publicity, fundraising, and corporate influence. In fact, critics say its primary purpose has become self-preservation. To this end, the pink ribbon culture functions to keep the breast cancer epidemic alive as a vital social problem while maintaining the impression that important work is being done to solve it. Although the swift current of pink ribbon culture quickly submerged the resistant ethos that galvanized much of the earlier movement, the persistent efforts of a counter-pink culture have always remained active. Later chapters will focus more completely on the countercurrents of pink ribbon culture, both at the level of cultural resistance and collective organizing. The selective history that follows shows how critical components of the breast cancer movement laid the groundwork for pink ribbon culture to materialize. These roots in advocacy provide continuity within the social history of breast cancer as part of the broader women's health movement, which lend legitimacy to pink ribbon culture without the more radical content.

Medical Consumerism

Medical consumerism is a term that refers to the belief that the users of health services should and do play an active role in making informed choices about their health.[8] The women's health movement of the 1970s emphasized the patient's right to accurate scientific and medical information to necessitate informed decision-making. Notably, the Boston Women's Health Book Collective developed *Our Bodies, Ourselves* in 1973 to empower women to educate themselves and other women about health issues. The book placed women's health in a radically new political and social context, which helped to launch and sustain the national and international women's health movements. The book permitted women for the first time to readily inform themselves about a wide range of health issues. By identifying and collaborating with individuals and health service organizations, it generated research and policy analyses and inspired women to become engaged in the political aspects of sustaining good health for themselves and their communities. Medical consumerism fostered a client-centered approach that was a springboard for organizing around the issue of breast cancer and prioritizing the perspectives of diagnosed women.

Journalist and activist Rose Kushner was committed to uniting the goals of breast cancer advocacy with the broader women's health movement. After being diagnosed with breast cancer in 1974 and researching her own disease, she became dedicated to the critical analysis of health issues, the rights of patients to access information and make choices, and the role of the medical consumer in shaping public policy. To further these goals, Kushner helped to establish the National Women's Health Network (NWHN) in 1975. The NWHN is an information clearinghouse and watchdog of federal policy on a variety of women's health issues. With regard to breast cancer, the organization has been concerned with the role of oral contraceptives and hormone therapy in breast cancer, the effects of cancer drugs, controversies surrounding mammography and conventional treatments, and aspects of the breast cancer industry that create barriers to improvements in women's health. For over three decades the network has been committed to social justice and a healthcare system that reflects the needs of diverse women.

In addition to her role in the NWHN, Kushner was a patient representative at the 1979 Consensus Conference of the National Cancer Institute on the surgical treatment of breast cancer. She was responsible for a landmark recommendation that changed the standard medical practice of performing both a biopsy and, if positive, a mastectomy immediately during the same surgery.[9] At that point radical mastectomies were still the norm, resulting in the removal of not only the breast and lymph nodes, but also the underlying chest muscle. Although it was the gold standard of breast cancer treatment well into the 1980s, the results were debilitating and produced no real health benefit for most women. The new process would separate the diagnostic biopsy from breast cancer treatment. Women would have the opportunity to get second opinions, consider treatment alternatives, and participate in the decision-making process *before* being treated. This change aligned with the broader mission of the women's health movement to uphold women's rights to make informed medical decisions.

Breast cancer organizing stressed a client-centered approach that required more cooperative doctor–patient interactions as well as information-sharing among diagnosed women. In 1977, the Self-Help Action Rap Experience (SHARE) in New York City was the first formal organization to offer mutual support programs from and to diagnosed women.[10] Y-ME, founded in Chicago in 1979, became the first national-level breast cancer organization, which provided educational programs, information on public policy, and hotline peer counseling by breast cancer survivors.[11] Rose Kushner also co-founded the National Alliance of Breast Cancer Organizations (NABCO) in 1986 with Diane Blum of Cancer Care, Nancy Brinker of the Susan G. Komen Breast Cancer Foundation, and Ruth Spear, a patient and author living in New York.[12] At its height, NABCO became a network of over 370 organizations, including advocates, institutions, and healthcare providers. These organizations helped to expand the breast cancer movement, reinforcing the idea that diagnosed women needed to be at the center of information assessment and social support.

As a key figure in the women's health and breast cancer movements, Rose Kushner especially emphasized a medical consumerist philosophy that recognized that information varied in quality and did not necessarily lead to the kind of knowledge that would save a person's life. She continually pointed out that empowered decisions could come only from the critical evaluation of evidence-based information. In her first book about breast cancer, *Breast Cancer: A Personal History and Investigative Report* (1975), Kushner's "autopathography" (i.e., an autobiography inspired by the influence of an illness or disability on the author's life) grew into a sustained investigative report on the status of breast cancer research and care in the United States and abroad.[13] Her second and third books, *Why Me: What Every Woman Should Know about Breast Cancer to Save Her Life* (1982)[14] and *Alternatives: New Developments in the War Against Breast Cancer* (1985),[15] addressed the medicalization of women through breast cancer treatment. The books laid a solid foundation for a breast cancer movement in which survivors-as-laypersons could develop enough critical knowledge about their disease and treatment to gain leverage not only in individual medical encounters but with the medical system as a whole. Kushner politicized the personal experience of breast cancer and lifted the veil surrounding the medical system's ineffectiveness and apparent lack of responsiveness to diagnosed women.

As the breast cancer movement continued to grow in the 1980s, the term *survivor* was used strategically to de-stigmatize the disease and to empower diagnosed women to take personal and collective action. Just as the survivors' movements against sexual violence used the survivor role to replace the role of victim,[16] the breast cancer movement used survivor discourse to promote women's empowerment and personal transformation, and to give voice to previously hidden personal experiences. The words and perspectives of breast cancer survivors emerged in support settings, public demonstrations, and personal accounts. As diagnosed women fulfilled the survivor role, many women's health activists promoted the kind of informed medical consumerism that Kushner encouraged.

With a few major exceptions, however, this critical stance started to erode. As pink ribbon culture took hold in the early 1990s, the survivor/medical consumer followed broader societal trends. The new medical consumerism was a form of mass consumption that involved tailoring one's choices to the available options, not questioning the options.[17] Attention to causes, alternatives, and other systemic issues was redirected toward the personal qualities of the medical consumer. The empowered breast cancer survivor was an optimistic medical consumer who had faith in medical science and conventional treatment.

Aesthetics and Normalization

In addition to opening up the discussion about breast cancer, the breast cancer movement promoted de-stigmatization through an aesthetic approach to coping. The aesthetic approach stressed the importance of restoring one's femininity following diagnosis and treatment, both physiarchly and socially. Normalizing women's experience through appearance and manner contributed to a model of survivorship that aligned both with the medical consumer model and traditional femininity. Doing so was a sign of victory in the war against breast cancer. This message circulated widely throughout fundraising and breast cancer awareness campaigns. Although many activists and organizations in the breast cancer movement rejected the aesthetic approach, it firmly took hold in the developing pink ribbon culture. A focus on "pink femininity" helped to construct a normalized identity for the breast cancer survivor that obscured the real impact of breast cancer on women and society.

The roots of normalization run deep. During much of the 20th century Victorian etiquette—including prudery, morbidity, sexism, and superstition—was a crucial force in keeping breast cancer hidden. Women's primary social function involved their sexual usefulness and family caretaking. Breast cancer was characterized to be a malady of the weaker sex, just another female problem that resulted from women's reproductive malfunctioning, negligence, sexual impropriety, or some other undisciplined behavior. Keeping such failures hidden helped to maintain the appearance of a fully functioning nuclear family. Since breast cancer was cast into a wide net of ailments related to women's deficient physical natures, it was relatively easy to bury it among menopause, fatigue, invalidism, and other female disorders of the time.[18] Existing patriarchal arrangements perpetuated the breast cancer taboo while it implicated women in causing their own affliction. Normalizing women's experiences of breast cancer was an attempt to bring the illness into the open and remove the blame.

The American Society for the Control of Cancer (ASCC), the precursor to the American Cancer Society, promoted public campaigns about breast cancer as early as the 1930s. Constructing breast cancer as a domestic war, the ASCC established the Women's Field Army (WFA) to encourage women to fulfill their responsibility to their families and communities here at home by sharing positive messages about breast cancer diagnosis and treatment with other women. With over 2 million women members at its peak, the large volunteer network "organized public events, canvassed neighbors and friends to raise money and generally spread the word about cancer."[19] Appealing to women's fear of getting the disease, the WFA became a formidable influence on public perceptions of breast cancer and women's role in the fight. The American Cancer Society disbanded the WFA in the early 1950s, but the cohesion among women who organized for the cause was a legacy that continued to shape American attitudes about breast cancer.[20] As one of the largest nonreligious charities, with powerful allies in private and public sectors, the American Cancer Society is still a primary source of information to the public about breast cancer.

The Reach to Recovery program, established in 1952, was the first mutual support activity for women with breast cancer that was oriented to aesthetics and normalization. Two women who were treated with Halsted radical mastectomies initiated the program to provide practical and emotional support to women who had had these disfiguring and frequently immobilizing surgeries. In 1969, the American Cancer Society adopted the program. Although women were fearful of getting breast cancer, there was mounting concern that women feared the dramatic mastectomy surgery to such a degree that they might avoid seeking medical attention if they found breast lumps. Reach to Recovery was designed to persuade women that breast cancer was not a disabling handicap.[21] The program focused on normalizing a woman's postsurgical appearance and promoting conciliatory behavior with the medical establishment. It provided temporary breast prostheses to enable women to conform to their wardrobes, and volunteers were survivors who would serve as walking evidence of medicine's ability to "cure" breast cancer. Reach to Recovery even forbade volunteers from discussing medical information to avoid contradicting doctors.[22]

Similarly, the "Look Good, Feel Better" program—developed by the Cosmetic, Toiletry, and Fragrance Association (CTFA) Foundation—assists women with their appearance following chemotherapy treatment, such as dealing with hair loss, dry skin, and brittle nails. Continuing its programmatic efforts to promote aesthetics and normalization, the American Cancer Society partnered with the CTFA Foundation in 1989 to provide a national network that would dispense information and access to the program. The National Cosmetology Association signed on as a third partner and encouraged its member cosmetologists to volunteer their services. "Look Good, Feel Better" programs exist in every state, the District of Columbia, and Puerto Rico, with products donated by 40 of the foundation's member companies.

In response to the gains of the women's health movement in resisting the constraints of gender and medicine, traditional feminine image and self-presentation became a touchstone for helping women to face breast cancer with greater confidence. Prosthetic breasts, wigs, makeup, and accessories masked the damage of breast cancer and contributed to an unblemished survivor identity. Instead of furthering the taboo related to women's innate frailty, traditional femininity would be cast as an empowering coping strategy. Having solidified once again the role of traditional femininity in relation to breast cancer, any woman who rejected the aesthetic approach was considered bad for morale.[23] By the 1990s, however, new organizations such as the San Francisco-based Breast Cancer Action and the Breast Cancer Fund actively rejected the aesthetic approach to draw attention to the effects of breast cancer on women's bodies, health, and life experiences.[24]

Despite these growing lines of dissent, traditional feminine aesthetics did help many breast cancer survivors to maintain a feminine appearance and an amiable impression. Since survivors are central to the breast cancer movement, the movement also made use of the aesthetic approach to cultivate a nonthreatening collective identity. Key figures within the breast cancer move- ment also had the political and economic clout to enhance the movement's credibility further. Samantha King points out that many of the women founders had high-status social positions that translated into social influence for their organizations:

> lawyers (e.g., Fran Visco, president of the National Breast Cancer Coalition), surgeons and researchers (e.g., Dr. Susan Love, founding member of NBCC), successful businesswomen (e.g., Amy Langer of the now defunct National Alliance of Breast Cancer Organizations), journalists (e.g., Rose Kushner), longtime political activists (e.g., Elenore Pred, founder of Breast Cancer Action), and lobbyists who understood the workings of the political and medical establishments.[25]

Being in the right social circles enabled these women in particular, and the movement in general, to increase their exposure, leverage, and access to financial resources.[26] Nancy Brinker's first Komen fund-raising event, for example, was held at a polo club, and (thanks to a call from a Texas real-estate magnate who was a friend of her husband's) former First Lady Betty Ford, who had had a mastectomy in 1974, was the guest of honor at the first annual Komen luncheon and a regular attendee thereafter.[27]

The legacy of high society and social influence unites with aesthetic norms to produce a social movement focused on image. The breast cancer luncheons, teas, galas, fashion shows, tennis and golf tournaments, and other elegant affairs grant social status to the movement while grounding it solidly in traditional femininity. Of course, traditional femininity stemming from the Victorian era is also white, heterosexual, and upper class. To open the breast cancer movement to more diverse membership, many organizations within pink ribbon culture have incorporated a public health model of cultural competency. This model encourages healthcare providers and organizations to make their practices more culturally and linguistically accessible. Ideally, the principles and activities of culturally and linguistically appropriate services should be integrated throughout an organization and undertaken in partnership with the communities being served.[28] Standards of cultural competency have contributed to an increase in the participation of African American, Hispanic, and Asian women in breast cancer organizing, and the visibility of diverse faces in pink ribbon culture.

However, breast cancer incidence and mortality rates reveal that race, ethnicity, class, and cultural differences continue to contribute to health disparities. African American women have a 10 percent lower incidence of breast cancer compared to white women, but they are more likely to die of the disease than women of other racial/ethnic backgrounds.[29] While the 5-year survival rate has improved overall (90 percent for white women), it has hovered around 77 percent for African American women for the past two decades.[30] To address the survival disparity, Komen launched its Circle of Promise in 2007, which focuses on increasing the involvement of African American women in its mission to raise more funds and to disseminate information about early detection to the African American community.[31] This focus is illogical, given that Komen reports that mammography rates are similar between African American women and white women (70 and 71 percent, respectively.) The program does not address the barriers that are most likely to contribute to the increased death rates for African American women, such as poverty, lack of access to quality healthcare or health insurance, delays in diagnosis follow-up and treatment, residence in communities with fewer breast care specialists, difficulty in accessing general preventive healthcare, increased exposure to environmental toxins, stress, and racial discrimination.[32] In addition, African American women may delay entry into the medical system for personal reasons such as concerns about providing for their families, or due to a history of mistrust of the healthcare system.

Despite greater representation of minority women (e.g., Komen's Circle of Promise boasts national representation from notable African American women such as René Syler and Synthia Saint James), the dominant discourses, cultural products, and broader socioeconomic and racial/ethnic composition of the mainstream breast cancer culture exert pressure to embody the traditional upper-class feminine aesthetic regardless of structural and cultural differences.[33] In her research of African American women's breast cancer organizing, LaShaune Johnson found a strong emphasis on "classyness" and sophistication in breast cancer programs and organizations run by African American women. She argues that these strategies are in part an attempt to prove the worth and trustworthiness of African American women to the social and cultural institutions that hold greater public status and power. Although the tea parties and golf tournaments held to raise money for African American patients resemble the events of pink ribbon culture, they can be just as alienating for many of the poor African American women who are beneficiaries.[34] Without changing the scripts of pink ribbon culture, the spirit of cultural competency manifests as surface-level adaptations to existing programs.

Similarly, breast cancer is the most commonly diagnosed cancer and the leading cause of cancer death among Hispanic/ Latina women. Despite increases in screening rates, these women still tend to be diagnosed at a later stage.[35] The 5-year survival rate for non-Hispanic Caucasian women with breast cancer is 85 percent, compared to 76 percent for Latinas. Poor health outcomes for this group of women are also related to structural barriers such as poverty, lack of insurance, low education levels, limited access to healthcare, negative provider attitudes, language differences, and sometimes citizenship. Cultural beliefs about modesty, family-centeredness, and fatalism may prevent open discussion of breast cancer.[36] To address language barriers, some organizations have made their breast cancer information available in Spanish. While this is a step toward cultural competency, community-based health organizations such as the Oakland-based National Latina Health Organization, founded in 1986, originally promoted needed services that may fall through the cracks when a person is ill, such as financial assistance for groceries, phone bills, transportation, and childcare. Such services seldom receive funding support from federal agencies or philanthropic foundations, yet they are fundamental to the reduction of health disparities among minority women.

Similarly, sexual minorities face cultural and structural barriers to healthcare and may have an overall risk for the development of breast cancer. Although there is limited epidemiological data on cancer rates in lesbians, results from the Women's Health Initiative found that the reported histories of breast cancers in postmenopausal women aged 50 to 79 were higher among lesbians compared to heterosexual women (7.1 percent and 4.9 percent, respectively).[37] Health care barriers for this population stem from misinformation about the health needs of lesbian and bisexual women,[38] poor access to care,[39] a general heterosexual focus among clinicians,[40] behavioral risk factors, and lower rates of participation in preventive health screenings such as routine gynecological services, birth control, and prenatal care.[41] In addition, women who partner with women are more directly affected by women's lower earning power compared to men and only rarely can benefit from their domestic partner's healthcare coverage that might pay for support and services. The Mautner Project, founded in 1990 following Mary-Helen Mautner's death from breast cancer, is dedicated to training healthcare providers about their lesbian patients and providing educational tools designed to foster improved health outcomes for lesbians. In cooperation with the Centers for Disease Control and Prevention, the Mautner Project developed the first and only culturally focused training program for physicians and healthcare staff on the healthcare needs of lesbians in an effort to aid providers in reaching their goal of serving underserved women.[42]

Throughout the breast cancer movement's history, perspectives about how best to empower diagnosed women have continually revealed a chasm between normalizing and exposing women's diverse experiences. Organizations within and beyond the movement have focused on revealing both the individual and systemic factors that affect breast cancer, including the unintended consequences of medical consumerism and the aesthetic approach to normalization. The counter-pink culture addresses systemic causes, structural barriers to care, scientific controversies, and the homogenization of women's experiences. The NBCC, for example, has emphasized universal quality healthcare since its inception. Yet the common image of the breast cancer survivor in pink ribbon culture overwhelmingly represents the normalizing feminine aesthetic—a survivor/medical consumer who is happy, whole, restored, and better than ever. Personal circumstances that do not fit the ideal are amalgamated into the dominant model or fall to the background. As Chapter 3 will show, the stigma that exists for breast cancer in pink ribbon culture is no longer the diagnosis, but the failure to present oneself as the aesthetically and emotionally pleasing breast cancer survivor.

A Cause of Epidemic Proportions, and the Rise of Pink October

In 1991, the Massachusetts Breast Cancer Coalition pressured the state to become the first in the nation to declare breast cancer an epidemic. This led to state monitoring of breast cancer incidence, increased breast cancer education and awareness activities, and financial investment in the disease. Organizers in Vermont lobbied successfully that same year for a bill requiring insurance companies to pay for mammograms, and in 1992 California created a state breast cancer research fund through an income tax check-off program and enacted laws guaranteeing standardized written information about breast cancer treatments for patients. Across the country, new breast cancer organizations were forming to push for social investment in the disease and a public commitment to promote policies that would lead to its eradication.

In the midst of growing concern about how to deal with increasing incidence rates and steady death rates, mammography came to signify awareness as well as responsible and proactive action on the part of public agencies and the informed and empowered medical consumer. National Breast Cancer Awareness Month (NBCAM), which was established in 1985 by the American Cancer Society with funding from the pharmaceutical company Zeneca Group plc, spread the message of early detection to save lives. Well-known public figure and breast cancer survivor Betty Ford helped to kick off NBCAM with an emotional televised appeal. Every October since then, NBCAM has been a platform for a variety of activities, products, and services related to breast cancer and mammography screening. During the 1993 NBCAM, President Clinton proclaimed the third Friday in October to be "National Mammography Day," encouraging companies, clinics, and radiologists to provide free or discounted screening on this special day.[43] After mammography was incorporated into insurance coverage and state and federal programs, screening as a prevention strategy would virtually guarantee continued investment in the cause. Coupled with public service campaigns, community events, news stories, and advertisements, NBCAM gave breast cancer a regularly occurring timeline for public outreach and cause promotion.

And then came the pink ribbon. According to an article in *MAMM* magazine, Komen started giving pink visors to breast cancer survivors running in its Race for the Cure in 1990. By the fall of 1991, the foundation had given pink ribbons to every participant in its New York City race. However, the ribbon was not introduced as the official symbol for breast cancer awareness until NBCAM in 1992. Evelyn Lauder of the Estée Lauder Companies, who was diagnosed with breast cancer in 1989, joined forces with then-editor of *Self* magazine to collaborate on a national breast cancer awareness campaign.[44] As a variation on the red HIV/AIDS ribbon, the pink ribbon set the stage for the strategic use of symbolism and mass media to influence public opinion and behavior as it related to breast cancer. Importantly, the pink ribbon reinforced the aesthetic approach to normalization that was important to the success of the breast cancer movement. The color pink evokes traditional femininity and the goodness and decency it conveys: emotionality, beauty, morality, and nurturance. By extension, the pink ribbon is an adornment that represents both a threat to traditional femininity and a virtuous and blameless illness.[45] Estée Lauder cosmetic counters distributed 1.5 million pink ribbons in 1992, accompanied by a laminated card describing proper breast self-examination.[46] The foundation that Lauder founded in 1993, the Breast Cancer Research Foundation, will have given out more than 85 million pink ribbons by the end of 2009.

The *pinking* of breast cancer readied the cause for mass dissemination and public consumption. October is now so closely identified with the cause of breast cancer that it is commonly referred to as "Pinktober," which is dedicated to "celebrating life, spreading awareness, and going pink in support of the fight against breast cancer."[47] Pinktober is upbeat, disseminates a general awareness message, encourages people to display (and therefore buy) pink products, and stresses the urgent and aggressive action inherent in any war metaphor. Later chapters will show how pink ribbon culture draws upon each of these dimensions to transmit key elements of the culture that keep the cause alive. NBCAM/Pinktober has been the springboard for transforming the cause into a national phenomenon with millions of supporters who raise billions of dollars to invest in a consumer-based version of breast cancer advocacy. According to Samantha King, breast cancer advocacy became an array of ubiquitous marketing strategies to consolidate the growth, financial assets, and political power of participating businesses and a few breast cancer organizations.[48]

Solidarity, Fundraising, and Publicity

The 1990s saw the emergence of new organizations, coalitions, and networks designed to address a range of breast cancer issues and policies. Many organizations continued to work toward providing emotional and practical support, identifying systemic causes of breast cancer, assessing medical treatments, analyzing policy, and/or evaluating conflicts of interest within the movement and the cancer industry. As breast cancer and the pink ribbon began to permeate corporate marketing strategies and a broad range of fundraising and advocacy activities, breast cancer culture started to take shape as a consumer-based culture. The mass distribution of pink ribbon symbolism and pink consumption began to favor the large-scale breast cancer organizations, as corporations strengthened their public relations packages through cause-marketing and corporate philanthropy.[49] Cause-marketing involves a marketing relationship between a corporation and a nonprofit organization for mutual benefit: the corporation sells products and gains consumer loyalty, and the nonprofit organization receives a portion of the proceeds. Increasingly, breast cancer organizations needed to decide whether to form partnerships with corporate sponsors.

Building on NBCAM and physical activity–based fundraising events, Susan G. Komen for the Cure (previously named the Susan G. Komen Breast Cancer Foundation) has become one of the largest nonprofit breast cancer organizations in the world. Growing from about 800 participants in Komen's first

5-kilometer "Race for the Cure" in 1983, the series expanded to over 1.5 million participants in 122 locations in the United States and 14 internationally.[50] In addition to huge numbers of participants, the races use over 100,000 volunteers. The Komen race series, coupled with other fundraising programs, educational initiatives, donations from individuals, and corporate partnerships, resulted in raising more than $275 million in revenue for the fiscal year ending March 1, 2007.[51] Komen had 94 official corporate partnerships in 2008, from Microsoft to General Mills to American Airlines to RE/MAX International. Whether purchasing computer software, cereal, air transportation, or real estate, consumers can donate to Komen indirectly through these corporations.[52] The foundation has invested $1 billion in community outreach programs to date.

Komen refers to itself as "a grassroots network" and claims to be "the voice" of the breast cancer movement. With 122 affiliate organizations to uphold the mother organization's mission, consumer-based strategies, and legislative agenda, Komen's directive to "Join the Global Breast Cancer Movement" equates Komen with that movement as well. With corporate partnerships and insider status, Komen's visibility, revenue, and strategic use of the pink ribbon helped to make the organization a major force in the developing pink ribbon culture. Komen, however, is not *the* voice of the breast cancer movement. There are other national, regional, state, and local organizations that provide the bulk of local services for diagnosed women and mobilize around diverse breast cancer issues.

In 1991, the NBCC was created as a national umbrella of over 600 organizations. In addition to its role in establishing the Department of Defense Breast Cancer Research Program in 1993, NBCC has ensured the program's annual funding increases, now totaling $2.1 billion. The coalition helped to expand access to healthcare through the Breast and Cervical Cancer Treatment Act (P.L. 106-354), which secured Medicaid coverage for low-income, uninsured women diagnosed with breast or cervical cancer through a federal program. It has been highly instrumental in persuading Congress to introduce bills related to consumer involvement, environmental cancer research, prescription drug coverage, genetic nondiscrimination in insurance, and the Patients' Bill of Rights. In addition to policy analysis, the coalition is committed to the importance of evidence-based medicine. To this end, the coalition evaluates scientific and medical information, develops position papers, and holds programs to educate the public on how to evaluate scientific and medical research. The coalition was ranked as one of the top 25 most influential groups in health policy in a University of Chicago survey, and it was the only grassroots organization, and the only breast cancer organization, to achieve that recognition.

When the NBCC was formed in 1991, it was Dr. Susan Love who was instrumental in mobilizing women from across the country. After an initial planning meeting that involved the Y-ME National Breast Cancer Organization, the Women's Community Cancer Project, Breast Cancer Action, Cancer Care, and Canact, there was an open meeting in Washington, DC.

Individuals from 75 organizations and representing a variety of interests started the organization. Focusing on the alliance among women survivors, the organizations involved were professional and grassroots, local and national, those exclusively focused on breast cancer and those addressing all cancers, physicians' groups, scientists, feminists, and others. Oriented to a network-based model, NBCC was committed to developing a broad-based coalition comprising member organizations that would also maintain their own distinct agendas for support, education, and advocacy.

Although Komen's founder, Nancy Brinker, was contacted for the initial planning meeting that started the NBCC, Komen was not listed among the organizations that attended,[53] nor did Komen become part of the board of directors. In fact, NBCC and Komen represent an ideological split in the national breast cancer movement about what constitutes beneficial content for breast cancer awareness and organizing activities and appropriate sources of breast cancer funding. NBCC has held to a medical consumerist model that focuses on patient empowerment through evidence-based medical decision-making. Maintaining a judicious stance with regard to the efficacy of current diagnostics and treatment, the lack of research into the causes of breast cancer, and loyalty to mammography screening despite scientific controversy surrounding its risks and benefits, NBCC holds a critical position in the movement and focuses on lobbying Congress for financial investment in breast cancer as a public health problem. In contrast, Komen's advocacy model relies on individual and corporate donations and sponsorships, and the foundation's advocacy arm, the Advocacy Alliance, focuses primarily on advancing policies that almost always relate to screening and increased public and federal investment in breast cancer.[54] While Komen gives strong advice, such as starting mammograms at age 40, there is no substantial analysis of the scientific controversies surrounding this agenda. (Chapter 5 includes a full discussion of the benefits and risks of mammography, its importance to the breast cancer industry, and the industry's ties to mainstream advocacy.)

In addition to NBCC and Komen, there are thousands of other organizations across the nation that are forgotten amid the flurry of pink ribbon culture. They shape breast cancer programs and support services in their own communities, advocate for patients' rights and quality care, raise their own funds, and advance cancer care legislation. The smaller community-based organizations generally use volunteer labor and obtain financial support from organization members, individual donations, local businesses, fundraisers, or grants from government agencies or other foundations, including Komen. These networks and organizations frequently provide the majority of local support services. Corporate interest in breast cancer since the early 1990s has made life for these organizations more tenuous: they struggle to secure their budgets, maintain their programs, and stay true to their missions.

NABCO closed its doors in 2004 after it became clear that the breast cancer community had become too crowded and focused on fundraising. A "Dear Friends of NABCO" letter announced the closing of the 18-year-old organization, commenting on an economic environment that is not conducive to organizations that provide labor-intensive programs such as case management.[55] NABCO's programs did not have the same allure as events and campaigns that involve the publicity-driven promotions so appealing to sponsors. The economic climate has forced organizations to choose: Align with the needs of the sponsors, or get out. The pink ribbon culture has also forced organizations to choose: Align with the dominant message, or [same outcome]. NABCO decided that self-perpetuation was not a worthy goal, and there was no need to give priority to fundraising instead of program delivery. Similarly, the organization conceded to the alleged mandate for a single voice on the issue of breast cancer.

To leverage their interests and resources, organizations in New York State formed a network of breast cancer organizations in 1998 to facilitate communication among organizations in the state, share information and programs, and create an organizing structure that could rival the economic climate and the pink ribbon culture. The New York State Breast Cancer Support and Education Network currently comprises 24 breast cancer–related service organizations and advocacy groups across the state, representing areas from Buffalo to Long Island. (The network's community-based organizations do not include Komen affiliates.)

Although the individual organizations maintain their own unique agendas for breast cancer support, education, and advocacy, the network assists member organizations through inter-organization referrals for services, programs, and resources. Another main function is to obtain regular consensus about its positions on legislative priorities and lobby the state legislature. Legislative priorities have included policies related to health insurance coverage and environmental issues related to cancer as well as broad and progressive policy issues, such as adopting the Precautionary Principle.

The Precautionary Principle states that in the absence of scientific consensus to the contrary, if an action or policy may cause severe or unalterable harm to the public or the environment, the burden of proof falls on those who are advocating the action or policy.[56] The principle suggests that there is a responsibility to intervene and protect the public from exposure to potential harm when scientific investigations discover a plausible risk. Progressive breast cancer organizations across the country have considered this principle to be a necessary step in mitigating and preventing environmental causes of breast cancer. Notably, the Breast Cancer Fund was formed in 1992 to advocate for the elimination of the environmental and other preventable causes of breast cancer. This group helped to pass a Precautionary Principle Purchasing Ordinance in San Francisco in 2005 and published the fifth edition of a comprehensive report analyzing the body of scientific evidence that links exposures to radiation and synthetic chemicals to an increased risk of breast cancer—*State of the Evidence 2008: The Connection Between Breast Cancer and the Environment*.[57] The Breast Cancer Fund has been an important organization in the development of an environmental breast cancer movement that rivals the dominant messages and organization of pink ribbon culture.[58]

In pink ribbon culture, the breast cancer movement is presented as "consensual." The large and visible impact of the large organizations, particularly Komen, creates the appearance that the movement is a cohesive, unitary force with an uncontested agenda. These organizations have created a political and socioeconomic structure that marginalizes other community-based organizations to varying degrees. The breast cancer movement is hardly consensual: its values, priorities, and strategies are negotiated and vigorously contested as organizations with diverse agendas evolve to advocate, educate, and provide support services. In addition to giving attention to a range of issues that are not addressed in the mainstream pink ribbon culture, many organizations outside of the pink mainstream follow the model of the National Women's Health Network and are less willing to accept funding from companies or organizations that may have a conflict of interest (e.g., those whose products or services include cancer diagnosis or treatment, or whose products may contribute to cancer incidence, such as pharmaceutical companies, chemical manufacturers, oil or tobacco companies, health insurance organizations, or cancer treatment facilities).[59] Against the tide of the pink culture, these organizations must find other ways to garner support and represent themselves.

UNINTENDED CONSEQUENCES

Breast cancer advocacy in the United States was crucial to the development of a breast cancer culture that is no longer limited to members of the movement or breast cancer survivors. Since the early 1990s, the elements of the breast cancer movement that shaped pink ribbon culture have been either diluted or intensified in service to its continued growth. As Chapter 4 will show, pink ribbon iconography has become the central feature, creating a representational relationship between the public and breast cancer. The rise in pink ribbon publicity has coincided with an increase in awareness and fundraising activities, collective mobilization, public and policy attention, and mammography screening. The primary function of pink ribbon culture is now to maintain breast cancer's status as a women's health epidemic, uphold the image that society is doing something about it, expand the social and political influence of key players in the breast cancer movement, and keep the money flowing.[60]

For some, the trade-off between pink spectacle and fundraising through cause-marketing is worth it. Larry Norton, MD, is the deputy physician-in-chief for breast cancer programs at Memorial-Sloan Kettering Cancer Center and medical director of the Evelyn H. Lauder Breast Cancer Center, housed in the same location. As one of the beneficiaries of the Evelyn Lauder Breast Cancer Research Foundation, which has generated more than $250 million since its founding, Norton argues that the proliferation of pink products offsets a federal research budget for cancer that is far too low (only $5 billion).[61] Similarly, the University of Texas M.D. Anderson Cancer Center is on track to receive $8 million over 8 years for the Morgan Welch Inflammatory Breast Cancer Research Program and Clinic, which American Airlines pledged through its Komen partnership. Inflammatory breast cancer is an aggressive breast cancer that represents 1 to 5 percent of diagnoses and has a 5-year survival rate of only 40 percent. According to the directors, the clinical trial developed from the grant will be the first line of treatment specifically targeting this cancer.[62]

There are no doubt other quality research projects that get their funding through cause-marketing programs. However, using breast cancer as a brand name has helped to divert public attention to "the Cause" and away from some of the key factors that are getting in the way of disease eradication.

First, each year, the American Cancer Society publishes facts and figures on cancer in the United States, including incidence and mortality. From 2000 to 2006, the number of invasive breast cancers (those that infiltrate the connective tissue and can invade blood vessels and lymph nodes) in women rose from 182,800 to 212,920 cases, and the number of non–life-threatening *in situ* cancers (early stage; those that have not invaded surrounding fatty tissues in the breast or spread to other organs) rose from 46,400 to 61,980 cases. The number of invasive cancers estimated for 2008 dropped to 182,460, while the number of *in situ* cancers continued to climb to 67,770.[63] Although death rates from breast cancer have decreased for white women since 1990, they have not decreased for African American women. Breast cancer remains the second leading cause of cancer death for all women (after lung cancer). The number of breast cancer deaths estimated each year from 2000 to 2008 has averaged 40,314 women, with small fluctuations up and down during this period.[64] The National Cancer Institute estimates that a woman in the United States has a 1 in 8 chance of developing invasive breast cancer during her lifetime; this risk was about 1 in 11 in 1975.

Although scientists have discovered some risk factors for breast cancer (such as age, reproductive factors, inherited genetic mutations, postmenopausal obesity, hormone replacement therapy, alcohol consumption, and previous history of cancer of the endometrium, ovary, or colon), the known risk factors account for only 30 percent of breast cancer cases. There are few interventions that reduce risk, and none of them prevent breast cancer.

Second, in much of pink ribbon culture, scientific controversies are avoided or simplified. For example, there is disagreement about the classification and best course of treatment for stage zero cancers, which are thought to be pre-cancers or risk factors. Lobular carcinoma *in situ* is controversial because it begins in the milk-producing glands but does not penetrate into the breast tissue. The classification of ductal carcinoma *in situ* as a breast cancer is under scrutiny because the condition does not tend to spread to other breast or organ tissues. In addition, chemoprevention drugs have questionable benefit. Major studies have shown that despite tamoxifen's ability to reduce breast cancer recurrence marginally in postmenopausal women, it increases the risk of uterine cancer. The majority of women who take the drug live no longer than women who do not take it.[65]

The most controversial issue involves the survival benefits of mammography. Mammography may not detect fast-growing malignancies early enough to affect cure; it leads to more aggressive treatment and unnecessary surgeries; and it offers only a modest benefit for women age 50 to 70 and a lesser benefit among women age 40 to 49.[66] Still, pink ribbon culture widely promotes mammography as the best weapon against breast cancer, fundamentally presenting it as a form of prevention, while omitting discussion of other causes and treatment-related breast cancer deaths.

There is increasing scientific evidence that exposure to common chemicals and radiation may contribute to the high incidence of breast cancer in the United States and worldwide. Pink ribbon culture omits, marginalizes, or downplays environmental factors, even though individual breast cancer advocates and grassroots breast cancer organizations have increasingly focused on the environmental links to breast cancer.[67] A study from the Silent Spring Institute in Cape Cod, which includes interviews with 56 grassroots organizational leaders in 27 states and two Canadian provinces, reports that 70 to 82 percent of leaders of breast cancer advocacy groups rated as "very important" research on workplace chemicals, air pollution, pesticides, household chemicals, drinking water, and endocrine-disrupting compounds. However, only 23 percent of these organizations are actively addressing environmental issues in their local communities.

Third, profit motives largely define pink ribbon culture within the context of a cancer industry that has many profit centers, including the pharmaceutical industry. As the nation's most profitable industry, Big Pharma uses advertising to exaggerate the benefits of their products, conceal risks, and expand their market base.[68] Chemotherapy drugs are highly profitable for both drug companies and doctors. Of Bristol-Myers Squibb's worldwide net sales of $5.1 billion in 2007, $1.5 billion came from wholesale distribution of oncology drugs.[69] Oncologists then profit from buying the drugs at wholesale and selling them to patients at marked-up prices. Financial reimbursement may have an effect on which chemotherapy drugs are prescribed to patients. More than half of all people diagnosed with cancer receive chemotherapy, even though "the benefits of chemotherapy are often fewer than we think."[70] While some women diagnosed with breast cancer will have increased survival with chemotherapy, many will not benefit from the treatment but will experience side effects, time lost from work, chemotherapy-related illness, a depleted immune system, and even treatment-related death. Those who receive radiation therapy are at a significantly higher risk of heart failure, especially if they are treated on the left side.[71]

Fourth, the status of breast cancer as the mother of all causes has situated breast cancer to be a choice illness for corporate cause-marketing. Now included in a variety of company portfolios, representing a range of different products and services, breast cancer has given companies and organizations greater economic advantage and public visibility. Typically, the concern about the cause-marketing relationship is about where the money is going: overhead costs versus program. To alleviate concern, the Komen foundation reports that it has been named "a top-rated charity by Charity Navigator, America's largest independent evaluator of charities, for a second year in a row." Komen does have a high rate of organizational efficiency: the organization spends about 83 percent of its revenue on program expenses, 10 percent on administrative expenses, and 7 percent on fundraising.[72] Komen relies on volunteerism, free or donated advertising, name recognition, corporate philanthropy, and corporate sponsorship to keep overhead low. But at what social cost?

Pink ribbon culture is built upon the early breast cancer movement that emerged from the 1970s and 1980s women's health movement and is sustained by mass publicity, the cancer industry, corporate and political interests, and a steady revenue stream. The culture extends a civic identity to those who support the fight against breast cancer (both individuals and corporations) through the consumption of pink ribbon products.[73] At this point a pink ribbon on any product or service signifies the good cause of breast cancer. Eradication of breast cancer is the headline, but when looking beneath the pink products and consumption practices, breast cancer as a social problem has become little more than a brand name with a recognizable pink logo. As Chapters 4 and 5 will demonstrate, survivors and supporters walk, run, and purchase for a cure as incidence rates rise, the cancer industry thrives, corporations claim responsible citizenship while profiting from the disease, and breast cancer is re-stigmatized for those who question or deny the pink ribbon model. With the goal of dominating the market, pink ribbon culture provides the organizational structure and cultural resources necessary to gain consumer loyalty and public trust while taking advantage of the good will and intentions of individuals who would like to do something about breast cancer.

Breast cancer advocacy continues to play an important role in maintaining pink ribbon culture. However, breast cancer advocacy has become embedded within a way of life that is oriented to breast cancer as a lifestyle. Grassroots activism remains, but it has been marginalized in a pink ribbon culture that draws on gender expectations, cultural scripts, consumption, and the persistent presence of mass media. Pink ribbon culture maintains the status of breast cancer as a women's health epidemic and the impression that key players in the culture are taking action to eradicate it. Without real advances toward the elimination of the disease, pink ribbon culture diverts attention to what people can do: get mammograms, participate in programs, and buy pink consumer goods. Such representations and symbolic actions often signify concern, promote solidarity, honor or memorialize someone, and even contribute some funds toward research or services. Yet they also obscure breast cancer survivors' actual experiences and the need for more resources and choices for those facing the disease; these actions limit other avenues for support and divert attention from deep analysis of the social and cultural forces that prevent the eradication of breast cancer.

NOTES

1. E. Leopold, A Darker Ribbon: Breast Cancer, Women, and Their Doctors in the Twentieth Century (Boston: Beacon Press, 1999), 214.

2. S. King, *Pink Ribbons Inc.: Breast Cancer and the Politics of Philanthropy* (Minneapolis: University of Minnesota Press, 2006); M. Klawiter, "Breast Cancer in Two Regimes: The Impact of Social Movements on Illness Experience," *Sociology of Health and Illness* 26 (September 2004): 845-74; P. Lantz & K. Booth, "The Social Construction of the Breast Cancer Epidemic," *Social Science & Medicine* 46 (1998): 907-18; Leopold, *A Darker Ribbon,* 204.

3. Leopold, *A Darker Ribbon,* 204.

4. *Ibid.,* 188-212. See also Boston Women's Health Collective, *Our Bodies Ourselves* (New York: Touchstone, 1976).

5. G. A. Sulik & A. Eich-Krohm. "No Longer a Patient: The Social Construction of the Medical Consumer," in *Advances in Medical Sociology, vol. 10: Patients, Consumers and Civil Society,* ed. S. Chambre and M. Goldner, 3-28 (Bingley, UK: Emerald Group Publishing, 2008).

6. King, *Pink Ribbons, Inc.,* xxxii.

7. Ibid.

8. J. Gabe, M. Bury, & M. A. Elston, *Key Concepts in Medical Sociology* (Thousand Oaks, CA: Sage, 2004), 217.

9. R. Kushner, *Breast Cancer: A Personal and an Investigative Report* (New York: Harcourt Brace Jovanovich, 1975).

10. SHARE. "About SHARE." http://www.sharecancersupport.org/about.php?path=none&pw=&lang=e&view=about. (Retrieved Dec. 1, 2008).

11. B. Brenner, "Sister Support," in *Breast Cancer: Society Shapes an Epidemic,* ed. A. Kasper and S. Ferguson (New York: Palgrave, 2000), 328-9.

12. U. Boehmer, The Personal and the Political: Women's Activism in Response to the Breast Cancer and AIDS Epidemic (New York: SUNY Press, 2000), 162.

13. Kushner, Breast Cancer: A Personal History.

14. R. Kushner, Why Me? What Every Woman Should Know about Breast Cancer to Save Her Life (New York: Saunders Press/Holt Reinhardt, 1982).

15. R. Kushner, Alternatives: New Developments in the War Against Breast Cancer (New York: Warner Books, 1985).

16. E. Bass & L. Thornton, I Never Told Anyone: Writings by Women Survivors of Child Sexual Abuse (New York: Harper Collins, 1991); T. McNaron & Y. Morgan, Voices in the Night: Women Speaking Out About Incest (Minneapolis: Cleis, 1982).

17. Sulik & Eich-Krohm, "No Longer a Patient."

18. Leopold, A Darker Ribbon.

19. D. Davis, *The Secret History of the War on Cancer* (New York: Basic Books. 2007), 117.

20. *Ibid.*, 129.

21. Brenner, "Sister Support."

22. Sharon Batt, *Patient No More: The Politics of Breast Cancer.* (Charlottetown, P.E.I., Canada: Gynergy Books, 1994).

23. Audre Lorde, *The Cancer Journals* (San Francisco: Aunt Lute Books, 1980/2006), 42.

24. Breast Cancer Fund, "Obsessed with Breasts" press release, ad campaign, January 2000.

25. King, Pink Ribbons, Inc., 108.

26. *Ibid.*, 109.

27. L. Belkin, "Charity Begins at ... The Marketing Meeting, The Gala Event, The Product Tie-In," *New York Times*, December 22, 1996, [section 6, p. 40].

28. The Office of Minority Health, "National Standards on Culturally and Linguistically Appropriate Services (CLAS)," 2009. http://www.omhrc.gov/templates/browse.aspx?lvl=2&lvlID=15 (accessed October 20, 2009).

29. W. E. Barlow, E. White, & R. Ballard-Barbash, "Prospective Breast Cancer Risk Prediction Model for Women Undergoing Screening Mammography," *Journal of the National Cancer Institute* 98 (2006): 1204-14.

30. American Cancer Society, "African American Cancer Facts and Figures for African Americans 2009-2010," http://www.cancer.org/downloads/STT/cffaa_2009-2010.pdf

31. Susan G. Komen for the Cure, "Susan G. Komen for the Cure Launches Circle of Promise Campaign," http://ww5.komen.org/KomenNewsArticle.aspx?id=7512 (accessed October 1, 2007).

32. R. G. Dean, "The Myth of Cultural Competence," *Families in Society* 82, no. 6 (2001): 623-30; D. Fassin, "Culturalism as Ideology," in *Cultural Perspectives on Reproductive Health, ed.* C. M. Obermeyer, 300-17 (Oxford: Oxford University Press, 2001); Y. Gunaratnam, "Culture Is Not Enough: A Critique Of Multi-Culturalism in Palliative Care," in *Death, Gender and Ethnicity,* ed. D. Field, J. Hockey, & N. Small, 166-86 (London: Routledge, 1997); Y. Park, "Culture as Deficit: A Critical Discourse Analysis of the Concept of Culture in Contemporary Social Work Discourse," *Journal of Sociology and Social Welfare* 32, no. 3 (2005): 11-33; J. Nelson & T. Macias, "Living with a White Disease: Women of Colour and Their Engagement with Breast Cancer Information," *Women's Health & Urban Life* 7 (2008): 20-39; Black Women's Health Imperative, "Black Women and Breast Cancer," Fact Sheet CFC #11148. (Washington, DC: Black Women's Health Imperative, 2009).

33. L. Cartwright, "Community and the Public Body in Breast Cancer Media Activism," *Cultural Studies* 12, no. 2 (1998): 117-38.

34. L. Johnson, "'A Really Elegant Affair': The Role of Class in African American Breast Cancer Organizations," [Paper Presented at] Eastern Sociological Society, Philadelphia, March 15-18, 2007.

35. J. W. Berg, "Clinical Implications of Risk Factors for Breast Cancer," *Cancer* 53 (1984): 589-91.

36. A. G. Ramirez, L. Suarez, A. McAlister, R. Villrreal, E. Trapido, G. A. Talavera, E. Perez-Stable, & J. Marti, "Cervical Cancer Screening in Regional Hispanic Populations," *American Journal of Health Behavior*, 24, no. 3 (2000):181-92; U.S. Department of Health and Human Services, "Racial and Ethnic Disparities in Health" (Washington, DC: DHHS, February 21, 1998); Latina Breast Cancer Agency, "Latinas: Breast and Cervical Cancer; "About Us." http://www.charityadvantage.com/ Latina_Breast_Cancer_AgencyFDXIDY/AboutUs.asp (2009).

37. A. L. Solarz, "Lesbian Health," *Current Assessment and Directions for the Future* (Washington, DC: National Academy Press, 1999); B. G. Valanis, D. J. Bowen, T. Bassford, E. Whitlock, P. Charney, & R. A. Carter, "Sexual Orientation and Health: Comparisons of the Women's Health Initiative Sample," *Archives of Family Medicine*, 9 (2000): 843-53.

38. J. V. Bailey, J. Kavanaugh, C. Owen, K. A. McLean, & C. J. Skinner, "Lesbians and Cervical Screening," *British Journal of General Practice* 50 (2000): 481-2.

39. D. J. Bowen, J. B. Bradford, D. Power, P. McMorrow, R. Linde, B. C. Murphy, et al., "Comparing Women of Differing Sexual Orientations Using Population-based Sampling," *Women and Health* 40 (2004): 19-34; A. L. Diamant, C. Wold, K. Spritzer, & L. Gelberg, "Health Behaviors, Health Status and Access to and Use of Health Care: A Population Based Study of Lesbian, Bisexual, and Heterosexual Women," *Archives of Family Medicine* 9 (2000): 1043-51.

40. E. J. Thompson, "Expressions of Manhood: Reconciling Sexualities, Masculinities, and Aging," *Gerontologist* 44 (2004): 714-8.

41. J. P. Brown & J. K. Tracy, "Lesbians and Cancer: An Overlooked Health Disparity," *Cancer Causes and Control* 19, no. 10 (2008): 1009-20; S. D. Cochran, V. M. Mays, D. Bowen, S. Gage, D. Bybee, & S. J. Roberts, "Cancer-Related Risk Indicators and Preventive Screening Behaviors among Lesbians and Bisexual Women," *American Journal of Public Health* 91

(2001): 591-7; A. K. Matthews, D. L. Brandenburg, T. P. Johnson, & T. L. Hughes, "Correlates of Underutilization of Gynecological Screening among Lesbian and Heterosexual Women," *Preventive Medicine* 38 (2004): 105-13.

42. Mautner Project: The National Lesbian Health Organization, "2008 Annual Report," http://www.mautnerproject.org/about_us/Annual_Reports/2008_MP_Annual_Report.pdf (October 25, 2009).

43. K. Miller, "AstraZeneca and Breast Cancer Advocacy," *Breast Disease* 10, no. 5-6 (1998): 65-70.

44. Enid Nemy, "At Work With: Evelyn Lauder; From Pink Lipstick To Pink Ribbons," New York Times, February 2, 1995, C1 (New York edition); S. Fernandez, "Pretty in Pink" (1998; repr. June/July 1998, MAMM); Business Wire, "SELF Magazine Celebrates 25th Anniversary in September 2004; A Generation of Healthy, Active Women Grew up Loving SELF," Business Wire, August 24, 2004, http://findarticles.com/p/articles/mi_m0EIN/is_2004_August_24/ai_n6166771 (accessed June 20, 2008); Estée Lauder, Inc., "Executive profiles: Evelyn H. Lauder," 2008, http://www.elcompanies.com/the_company/evelyn_h_lauder.asp (accessed June 20, 2008).

45. B. K. Rothman, "Genetic Technology and Women," in *Women, Gender, and Technology*, ed. M. F. Fox, D. G. Johnson, & S. V. Rosser, 111-21 (Urbana and Chicago: University of Illinois Press, 2006).

46. Fernandez, "Pretty in Pink."

47. "Pinktober," [Blog] http://www.pinktober.org/ (accessed October 1, 2009).

48. J. A. Fosket, C. Karran, & C. LaFia, "Breast Cancer in Popular Women's Magazines from 1913-1996," in *Breast Cancer: Society Shapes an Epidemic*, ed. S. Ferguson & A. Kasper, 303-24 (New York: Palgrave, 2000); King, *Pink Ribbons, Inc.*; Klawiter, "Breast Cancer in Two Regimes."

49. King, Pink Ribbons, Inc.

50. Susan G. Komen for the Cure©, http://ww5.komen.org/AboutUs/InternationalRaces.html (accessed October 15, 2009).

51. Susan G. Komen for the Cure©, "2006-2007 Final Audited Financial Statements," http://ww5.komen.org/AboutUs/FinancialInformation.html (accessed December 8, 2008).

52. Susan G. Komen for the Cure©, "Corporate Partners," http://ww5.komen.org/CorporatePartners.aspx (accessed December 8, 2008).

53. Susan Love with Karen Lindsey, *Dr. Susan Love's Breast Book*, 4th ed. (Cambridge, MA: Perseus Books, 2005, fully revised), 588-92.

54. Susan G. Komen for the Cure Advocacy Alliance, "Our Positions," http://www.komenadvocacy.org/content.aspx?id=58 (accessed October 25, 2009).

55. Eric T. Rosenthal, "The Closing of NABCO," *Oncology Times* 26, no. 5 (March 2004): 24, 27.

56. C. Raffensperger & J. Tickner, eds., Protecting Public Health and the Environment: Implementing the Precautionary Principle (Washington, DC: Island Press, 1999).

57. J. Gray, ed., Breast Cancer Fund. 2008. State of the Evidence 2008: The Connection between Breast Cancer and the Environment, 5th ed. (San Francisco: Cooperative Printing, 2006).

58. B. Ley, From Pink to Green: Disease Prevention and the Environmental Breast Cancer Movement (New Brunswick, NJ: Rutgers University Press, 2009).

59. Breast Cancer Action©, "Policy on Corporate Contributions," http://bcaction.org/index.php?page=policy-on-corporate-contributions (accessed November 25, 2008).

60. B. Ehrenreich, "Welcome to Cancerland: A Mammogram Leads to a Cult of Pink Kitsch," *Harper's Magazine* (Nov. 2001): 43–53. Klawiter, "Breast Cancer in Two Regimes; King, *Pink Ribbons, Inc.*

61. M. Frazier, "ing Pink," *deltaskymag.com*, October 2009, 59-65.

62. American Airlines, "Inflammatory Breast Cancer Already Making Gains in First Year of Funding," http://www.aa.com/i18n/specialty-Pages/komen_IBCPromiseGrant.jsp (accessed October 15, 2009).

63. American Cancer Society, Cancer Facts and Figures, 2007; Cancer Facts and Figures, 2006; Cancer Facts and Figures, 2005; Cancer Facts and Figures, 2004; Cancer Facts and Figures, 2003; Cancer Facts and Figures, 2002; Cancer Facts and Figures, 2001; Cancer Facts and Figures, 2000 (Atlanta, ACS, various years).

64. Ibid.

65. Love, *Dr. Susan Love's Breast Book*; M. De Gregorio & V. Wibe, *Tamoxifen and Breast Cancer* (New Haven, CT: Yale University Press, 1994).

66. Peter C. Gotzsche & Ole Olsen, "Is Screening for Breast Cancer With Mammography Justifiable?" *Lancet* 355 (January 8, 2000, updated 2001): 129-34; Ole Olsen & Peter C. Gotzsche, "Cochrane Review on Screening for Breast Cancer with Mammography," *Lancet* 358, no. 9290 (2001): 1340-2, http://image.thelancet.com/extras/fullreport.pdf

67. Silent Spring Institute, "Grassroots Breast Cancer Advocacy and the Environment: A Report on Interviews with Grassroots Leaders" (Newton, MA: Silent Spring Institute, 2005), www.silentspring.org/newweb/activists/index.html.

68. According to the *Prescription Drug Trends* [www.kff.org, "2008 Drug Fact Sheet" (accessed October 10, 2009)] report published by the Kaiser Foundation, "spending for consumer advertising in 2007 was over 4 times the amount spent in 1996 ($3.7 billion vs. $0.8 billion)." The report also identifies the pharmaceutical industry as the nation's most profitable from 1995-2002, and among the top five profitable industries from 2002-2007.

69. Bristol-Meyers Squibb, Product Sales Summary, "2007-2008 Product Sales Summary," http://investor.bms.com/phoenix.zhtml?c=106664&p=irol-sales (accessed December 10, 2008; Rehema Ellis,

"Cancer Docs Profit From Chemotherapy Drugs," *NBC News*, Sept. 21, 2006. Congressional Record.

70. Love, Dr. Susan Love's Breast Book, 382.

71. J. Cuzick, H. Stewart, L. Rutqvist, et al., "Cause-Specific Mortality in Long-Term Survivors of Breast Cancer Who Participated in Trials of Radiotherapy," *Journal of Clinical Oncology* 12 (1994):447-53; G. Gagliardi, I. Lax, & L. E. Rutqvist, "Partial Irradiation of the Heart," *Seminars in Radiation Oncology* 11 (2001): 224-33.

72. Charity Navigator©," Susan G. Komen for the Cure: Working to Save Lives and End Breast Cancer Forever," http://www.charitynavigator.org/index.cfm?bay=search.summary&orgid=4509

73. King, Pink Ribbons, Inc.

THREE

MIXED METAPHORS
War, Gender, and the Mass Circulation of Cancer Culture

*Cancer is war. I knew I needed to arm myself to fight
this disease. My strategy was to attack it from four different
angles…physical…spiritual…emotional…mental…Right now
my negativity is in remission, and it's a constant battle to remain
a healthy optimist.*

MARISA ACOCELLA MARCHETTO, CANCER VIXEN[1]

The war on breast cancer has been raging throughout the
20th century. The 1936 the Women's Field Army (WFA)
of the American Society for the Control of Cancer (ASCC)
advertised the weapons and tactics of war. The WFA operated
with a military structure that was "organized vertically, complete with an officer corps and foot volunteers. Members wore
brown uniforms with insignia of rank" and enlisted women on
behalf of their families and communities.[2] The mission was to
encourage women to participate willingly and enthusiastically in
regular screening and conventional breast cancer treatment,
while cancer propaganda promoted fear, presented medical science and research as the best weaponry, and generally inspired
loyalty to the war. Imagery and language such as the *sword of hope,*

arsenal of information, and *trench warfare* in the *attack* against breast cancer charged women with the responsibility to use these weapons if they wanted hope for a cure. The WFA used traditional gender expectations about women's intrinsic nurturing abilities and responsibilities to provide care for others to encourage women's participation in the volunteer army.[3] In 1945 the ASCC reorganized to become the American Cancer Society. World War II was over and the American Cancer Society saw an opportunity to re-energize the war on cancer as the enemy at home.

Words such as *fight, battle,* and *war* commonly describe the relationship between those on the side of the diagnosed (soldiers, armies) and cancer itself (enemy, beast, and predator). The American Cancer Society and its precursor the ASCC successfully used war rhetoric to mobilize public opinion and raise awareness about cancer and cure. Medical doctor Baron Lerner traces the strategic use of war metaphor in *The Breast Cancer Wars.*[4] He argues that the concept of war in breast cancer's early social history had powerful effects on public opinion, political influence, medical practices, and the personal experience of breast cancer. Forcing sides in the war enabled the emergent cancer culture to blame women who did not engage properly in battle (i.e., aggressively using the weaponry of breast examination and medical science). Lerner identifies examples from the 1940s and 1950s of physicians and popular health magazines that castigated women who did not follow the commands of medical authorities. A callous statement from a medical surgeon described the woman who did not seek screening and treatment as having "committed suicide almost as certainly as if she had blown out her brains with a pistol."[5] Such illustrations in the early war on breast cancer positioned medical men (with scientific weaponry) as the commanders and saviors of women. Today, war imagery and terminology continue to dominate the cancer lexicon and structure social responses to the disease.

The war on cancer, like any war, is an uncertain state of affairs. Anthropologist Mary Douglas[6] argues in *Purity and Danger* that ambiguity is a source of powerful symbolism. Societies perceive uncertainty to be so dangerous that they develop complex classification systems to recast ambiguous situations into something clear-cut and manageable. The use of war metaphor is a symbolic attempt to demystify the uncertainty of cancer by categorizing it into a simple value system. The war metaphor draws upon binary categories such as good/evil, brave/cowardice, strong/weak, and victor/victim. Because one set of characteristics is more socially valued than the other, the binary system differentiates what is socially appropriate from that which is socially inappropriate. In the war on cancer goodness, bravery, strength, and victory are more highly valued than badness, cowardice, weakness, and defeat. In this way the binary system helps to establish symbolic consensus about how to deal with cancer, creating assurance in the face of uncertainty. The binary categories used in the war metaphor also operate in conjunction with a broader classification system.

Douglas argues that rituals, myths, poems, and other cultural processes use binary categories to create the classification system and thereby focus experience. Valued categories exist in opposition to devalued categories and in relation to one another. According to Douglas societies generally value the normal, healthy, and pure more highly than the abnormal, unhealthy, or polluted. Many modern societies also value the masculine more highly than the feminine. A simple nursery rhyme about "what little girls are made of" associates femininity with the characteristics of "sugar" (softness), "spice" (emotion), and "everything nice" (an ethic of caring). The classification system automatically constructs masculinity in opposition, equating boys and men with the socially valued characteristics of toughness, rationality, and dominance. Not only are women defined to be the weaker sex, the feminine characteristics of emotionality and nurturance falter beneath the masculine pursuit of rationality and power. Because the system is relational, valued characteristics confer worth to other valued characteristics and vice versa. The masculine gains status through association with the normal, healthy, and pure whereas the feminine loses status by association with the opposite traits. Social institutions and processes seamlessly maintain the binary system by incorporating and normalizing gender expectations and stereotypes.[7]

The prioritization of masculine rationality over feminine emotionality has a long history that centers on a philosophy that views the body as separate from the mind and spirit, or a *mind–body dualism*. René Descartes (1596–1650) was famous for his doctrine of dualism, according to which the mind and the body are two entirely distinct types of substances.[8] Descartes proposed that bodies are material substances that can and will ultimately disintegrate, whereas the mind is immaterial and not subject to decay. The Cartesian philosophy identifies the mind with the rational and immortal soul, and the human body as a machine that can be analyzed in terms of its parts (i.e., anatomy and physiology). The mind–body dualism had a major impact on Western thinking and, in turn, Western medicine. The adage "mind over matter" shapes common-sense ideas about the role of personality and emotion in determining physical realities, and reinforces the idea that the body should be controlled and disciplined. Controlling emotion so that it serves rational decision-making and bodily control implicates a gender system that equates the feminine with embodied emotion and the masculine with disembodied rationality.

When facing a cancer diagnosis, the desire for assurance draws on the binary classification system to recast the uncertainty of illness to something more manageable, and more valued. Because of the salience of gender, the conceptual categories that operate within the war metaphor use the classification of masculine/feminine to restore a semblance of normalcy. The broader cancer culture in the United States assimilates the already existing system to create a divergent masculine/feminine ethos. The pink ribbon culture then rearticulates the masculine/feminine ethos to create a unique model of breast cancer survivorship.

THE MASCULINE AND FEMININE ETHOS OF AMERICAN CANCER CULTURE

The war on cancer is a dramatic rhetorical struggle as competing agents try to shape the language, beliefs, and experiences of cancer. The masculine ethos is most prevalent, aligning with imagery of victorious heroism, sporting competition, and the war metaphor.[9] A competing feminine ethos resists the war metaphor in favor of nurturance, empathy, and a relational orientation. Two powerful organizations represent ideal types of these competing gender cultures, the LIVE**STRONG** Lance Armstrong Foundation, founded in 1997, and Gilda's Club, started in memory of Gilda Radner in 1991.[10] Both organizations support multiple types of cancers and use celebrity power to raise awareness and financial support for their programs and advocacy. They have also developed initiatives designed to have a vital impact on public health policy, support services, and the culture of cancer in the U.S. and worldwide. However, the two organizations differ in their use of masculine and feminine characteristics to further their respective visions of cancer survivorship.

LIVESTRONG and the Masculine Ethos

The LIVE**STRONG** Lance Armstrong Foundation represents the masculine ethos of survivorship in American cancer culture.

Cyclist Lance Armstrong, the unprecedented seven-time winner of the Tour de France, secured six of these wins after receiving aggressive treatment for testicular cancer that had metastasized to his brain and lungs. Even before his treatment ended, Armstrong started the LIVE**STRONG** charity cancer foundation in his name to inspire and empower people affected by cancer. Armstrong's illness identity characterizes the organization and emphasizes the importance of facing cancer with aggressiveness, dominance, rationality, and especially strength.[11]

The foundation's name, the LIVE**STRONG** Lance Armstrong Foundation (original emphasis), encapsulates the role of strength in Armstrong's vision of survivorship. The word "strong" in upper-case bold lettering is then repeated in its founder's surname, Armstrong. The word is again reiterated on the yellow plastic fundraising wristbands that are imprinted with the words "LIVE STRONG" and on a variety of products for sale on the foundation's website. Armstrong's cancer biography also emphasizes strength and fully concretizes an illness identity that incorporates the masculine ethos of survivorship. To illustrate, I include excerpts of "Lance's Story" as it is featured on the foundation's public website:[12]

> At age 25, Lance Armstrong was one of the world's best cyclists. He proved it by winning the World Championships, the Tour Du Pont and multiple Tour de France stages. Lance Armstrong seemed invincible and his future was bright. Then they told him he had cancer. Next to the challenge he now

faced, bike racing seemed insignificant. …Like most young, healthy men, Lance ignored the warning signs, and he never imagined the seriousness of his condition. Going untreated, the cancer had spread to Lance's abdomen, lungs and brain. His chances dimmed.

Proving that one is a champion through a list of wins is to be expected in the world of professional sport. However, the competitiveness, aggressiveness, and dominance that sporting language also illustrates typify idealized masculine traits. The champion who appears to be invincible is the manliest man of all, at least until illness calls this status into question. To avoid emasculation, Armstrong (the man) is equated with the masculine characteristics of the category of *young, healthy men* who are tough enough to avoid pain.

Even though Armstrong's bright future was dimmed with a serious cancer diagnosis, his story goes on to further demonstrate how his masculinity enabled him to take charge of his illness experience and win. Reiterating the importance of competition, Armstrong's story expresses the masculine expectations for initiative, control, rationality, and performance.[13]

Then…physical conditioning, a strong support system and competitive spirit took over. He declared himself not a cancer victim but a cancer survivor. He took an active role in educating himself about his disease and the treatment. Armed with knowledge and confidence in medicine, he underwent aggressive treatment and beat the disease.

Armstrong refuses victimization and from a position of power takes on a survivor identity. With Armstrong as the role model, cancer survivorship then takes on the characteristics that this identity emphasizes. War language further reinforces rational action, as Armstrong aggressively arms himself with information to prepare for battle and declare victory.

The foundation also uses the war metaphor in its national campaign to recruit a *LIVESTRONG Army* to *fight* cancer.[14] Armstrong's rallying call is a response to the 2006 federal cutback to the National Cancer Institute, the first reduction in 30 years. Reminiscent of the WFA discussed earlier, war language suggests urgency and the directive to line up to take appropriate action. War metaphor defines the situation as an emergency in which no sacrifice is excessive.[15] The masculine ethos would have women and men becoming soldiers, enlisting in war, following the direct orders of the medical commander(s)-in-charge, and submitting to the collateral damage of aggressive methods of treatment.

Lance's story ends with the creation of his cancer foundation and position as the self-appointed leader of cancer survivorship, both as an *advocate* and a *world representative.*

> During his treatment, before his recovery, before he even knew his own fate, he created the Lance Armstrong Foundation. This marked the beginning of Lance's life as an advocate for people living with cancer and a world representative for the cancer community…He plans to lead this fight, and he hopes

that you join him. This is a life he owes to cancer. This is his choice to live strong.

Armstrong describes his life as beholden to cancer, which is the impetus for his choice to live strong and lead others into battle. His desire to shape cancer culture in his own image is as clear as his story: to be an exemplary survivor, individuals must be strong and determined, take rational action, engage in battle, have faith in medicine, and win.

Armstrong and his foundation have received widespread support. After winning seven Tours and a host of other cycling races, Armstrong garnered extensive media attention and had an enormous following. He wrote two books about his experience (*It's Not about the Bike* in 2000 and *Every Second Counts* in 2003) that highlight his cycling career, his cancer biography, and his personal life.[16] Armstrong's celebrity profile and illness identity have had a visible public impact, which have enabled him to parlay his social status into mass support for the foundation: in 2006 LIVE**STRONG** had over $50 million in net assets, $35.7 million in net revenues and other support, and nearly 138,000 volunteer hours for program services and fundraising campaigns.[17] The success of the foundation has been a vehicle for Armstrong to affect both cancer culture and public policy. In doing so, he continues to fashion an illness identity that strengthens the masculine ethos of survivorship.

Armstrong's book co-author, Sally Jenkins, is a writer for the *Washington Post* sports section. She wrote an article in the *Post* in 2008 that addressed Armstrong's ambitions.[18]

> The man's…got big plans: In addition to licking cancer, he may want to run for governor in Texas some day…In 2007, Armstrong went on a USO tour of Iraq and Afghanistan, and campaigned hard for a Texas state measure, Proposition 15, to appropriate up to $3 billion for the Cancer Prevention and Research Institute of Texas. It's the largest state anti-cancer funding program ever, and when it passed he called it a bigger rush than he ever had winning the Tour.

Manly men like Armstrong get a *rush* from success and challenge. Whether physical or social, the rush increases when dominating the opponent. In this brief segment of Jenkins' article, the words *big, bigger,* and *largest* get this message through. Armstrong dominates. He beat cancer; he won the Tour, and if he wants to hold political office, he'll do that too. This humble researcher and avid fan imagines that Armstrong has honorable intentions. But just as winning the Tour was "not about the bike," Armstrong's war on cancer is not just about cancer.

Masculine ideals encourage men to render their illnesses invisible, or heroically transform them into social capital.[19] Armstrong has done both. In sharing his cancer biography publicly, he paints a portrait of himself that acknowledges his cancer diagnosis and treatment while obscuring its reality beneath heroism and an almost inhuman capacity. This story resonates with socially dominant masculine ideals. The website AskMen. com states: "Any guy that wants to educate the public about a disease that he was still battling at the time deserves our admiration. This man had cancer in his brain and lungs, but fought back to become No. 1 in his sport."[20] In demanding that the male audience admire Armstrong, the writer insists on collective social recognition for the masculine illness identity that Armstrong represents. Its message marks Armstrong's efforts as heroic, admirable, and attainable for any man who exhibits the characteristics that he did. However, just as Jenkins's article emphasized, only triumphant men deserve high status and public admiration. This separates Armstrong from the lesser men who perhaps did not fight adequately enough to win.

For Armstrong and his foundation, veneration forms the basis of a web of social networks oriented to his mission and his message. The masculine ethos of survivorship aligns with traditional masculinity such that any man who takes on these characteristics can be manly and fight cancer at the same time. The masculine ethos typically controls the terms of engagement in U.S. cancer survivorship. Because the masculine ethos is generalized, the reader is left to assume that women should respond to cancer in similarly masculine ways. Many women feel compelled to do so. However, there is a feminine ethos in the cancer culture that seeks to cope differently.

Gilda's Club and the Feminine Ethos

Just as norms of masculinity characterize the LIVE**STRONG** model of cancer survivorship, traditional femininity typifies the feminine ethos of cancer survivorship. Stressing nurturance, empathy, and a relational orientation, Gilda's Club is a cancer support organization named in memory of comedian Gilda Radner that exemplifies the feminine ethos. Radner died from ovarian cancer at age 42. She was best known for her work on NBC's *Saturday Night Live*, and she also wrote a biography that describes her life with cancer, *It's Always Something*. Gilda's Club is a network of affiliate clubhouses where men, women, and children of all ages living with all types of cancer, as well as their friends and families, learn how to live with cancer. The name of the organization originated from a statement Radner once made that cancer gave her "membership to an elite club [she]'d rather not belong to."[21] This message reflects Radner's awareness that cancer, like any other club, has rules of social engagement. However, Radner also believed that cancer was an individual experience for which the typical rules were inadequate.

The Gilda's Club philosophy of cancer survivorship runs counter to the masculine ethos of the LIVE**STRONG** model. The organization uses a feminine ethos to create an alternative way of living with cancer that omits the war metaphor, recognizes the limitations of conventional models, and promotes community-building, shared experience, and respect for the diverse ways of living with cancer. The specific mission of Gilda's Club is to increase the understanding that cancer does not occur in isolation, but within the family and social networks of individuals. The organization argues that emotional and social support are just as important as medical care, and intentionally holds lectures, workshops, and social events in a homelike setting.[22] The club also supports the idea that cancer is a personal experience. The *It's Always Something Room*, named after Radner's biography, is designated as a "quiet place for personal refuge." Prioritizing respect for the many personal approaches to living with cancer, the feminine ethos challenges the notion that a single metaphor is sufficient to understand the meaning and experience of cancer.

The organization's feminine ethos offers an alternative way of talking about and dealing with cancer. Gilda's Club International has consciously created a new cancer lexicon, and its Web site includes a section dedicated to "Gilda's Club Language."[23] In addition to words such as "community," "warm," "welcoming," and "a place to express a full range of feelings," Gilda's Club deliberately avoids words that, they believe, "convey or reinforce misconceptions about cancer."[24] The organization provides a list of its own examples, such as the following:

People living with cancer—NOT—Cancer victims or patients
Learning to live with cancer—NOT—Coping with cancer or facing a life-threatening illness
Regaining control & well-being—NOT—Doing battle, struggling with cancer, or fighting for recovery

The notion of *living* with cancer, rather than *coping,* is similar to Armstrong's message when he refuses to call himself a cancer *victim* and instead chooses to live *strong.* While the masculine ethos emphasizes a form of strength that is fortified with war imagery, Gilda's Club denounces the war metaphor and stresses *control* and *well-being.*

Similar to LIVE**STRONG**, which is characterized in terms of Armstrong's story and masculine message, Gilda's Club promotes a feminine illness identity through Radner's story and feminine message. The use of Radner's first name in the Club's title draws attention to the informality typically associated with a feminine relational orientation. In the binary classification system, formality is acceptable and publicly prescribed, whereas informality represents that which is private, illicit, and unofficial. Because the institutionalized gender system symbolically assigns women to the private sphere and men to the public, the association of women with informal behavior and relations sustains the notion that women are not to be taken seriously. When coupled with Radner's career in comedy, the feminine illness identity she represents takes on an air of triviality, even as Armstrong's illness identity—compatible with masculine norms and his career as a professional athlete—is both serious and socially sanctioned.

The commentary on the back cover of *It's Always Something* reiterates Radner's informality and emphasizes her traditional feminine attributes:

> The voice is pure Radner, part determined superwoman, part loveable brash child, and part generous-hearted comic offering inspiration and hope.[25]

Radner represents the class of superwomen who successfully handle several different roles such as marriage, motherhood, and career. The generosity, inspiration, and hope that she offers to others illustrate a feminine ethic of nurturance. At the same time, having played a little girl in some of her comedy routines, the description can't help but infantilize her as an impetuous child, while condemning her emotionality.

The illness identities described through the examples of Armstrong and Radner illustrate how gender and illness combine to construct a gendered illness identity that is then presented as universal in American cancer culture. Associating traditionally masculine or feminine characteristics with rhetoric that is intended to empower the public toward a specific mode of survivorship enables the existing gender system to reinforce as well as obscure the masculine/feminine ethos. Because masculinity is socially valued in the binary system, a man who follows Armstrong's example will fight cancer heroically and admirably, with strength, perseverance, and victory, without compromising his masculinity; in fact, choosing the masculine ethos will increase his social capital. On the contrary, a woman who chooses the LIVE**STRONG** masculine ethos must transgress gender boundaries to do so successfully. The masculine ethos demands that individuals suppress emotion and a relational orientation, while taking a competitive and aggressive stance. Because the masculine ethos is highly valued, however, even women will garner social capital in the attempt.

Those who reject the LIVE**STRONG** model and are willing to accept a devalued feminine ethos may turn to Gilda's Club for an alternative approach to cancer survivorship. Because femininity is socially devalued in the binary system, men who prefer the feminine ethos of survivorship risk demasculinization. On the other hand, women who do so are able to present themselves in ways that adhere to traditionally feminine expectations.

Through processes of socialization, individuals learn consciously and unconsciously what is expected of them in their cultural environments and how to behave accordingly. A cancer diagnosis is a major disruption that causes individuals to enter a cultural environment that is often foreign to them. The desire to restore normalcy encourages them to adopt an existing mode of survivorship. The cancer culture in the United States presents two options, a masculine or feminine ethos. Based in a binary gender system, these alternatives rely on traditional gender expectations to construct a vision of survivorship that makes sense on a symbolic level. The powerful organizations that promote these divergent philosophies convey them through the gendered illness identities of the celebrities for whom they are named. In carving out its own unique cancer culture, pink ribbon culture incorporates elements of both the masculine and feminine ethos while highlighting a specific version of femininity that is colored pink.

PINK FEMININITY

The color *pink* has been a socializing agent since the 1940s to prepare women for their roles in American society and naturalize gender-stereotyped views of the world. Pink and blue imagery are clearly visible in early childhood socialization. However, socialization occurs throughout the course of a person's life—from early childhood to adulthood, and whenever individuals develop a new sense of self, develop habits, take on new roles, and learn (relearn) how to get along in different social groups and cultural environments. Numerous cultural inputs influence the ongoing gender socialization process. Representing traditional feminine norms and values within the binary gender system, the color pink shapes gender ideology. Over time, a popularized form of gender ideology has developed into what I call *pink femininity*. Cultural representations of pink femininity convey the softness, innocence, dependence, and virtue of girlhood and true womanhood while simultaneously symbolizing the threatening qualities of independence, cunning, and manipulative seduction. The subtle and consistent nature of pink femininity throughout American culture provides the backdrop for pink ribbon culture, which incorporates pink femininity into its media messages and cultural representations to convey its messages of breast cancer support, awareness, and survivorship.

Mass media has been an important agent of gender socialization and cultural production in the development of pink femininity. Lynn Peril's cultural history *Pink Think*[26] analyzes popular culture from the 1940s to the 1970s and shows how advertising and advice experts fashioned a feminine ideal packaged in pink. *Girls* were presented as soft, pure, impressionable, and pretty, yet they were also depicted as sly, mysterious, and prone to tantrums. In turn, the *women they would eventually become* were duplicitously cast as moral, emotional, empathetic, and nurturing as well as seductive, manipulative, and secretive. For girls and women, physical attractiveness and good beauty habits were crucial, and it was never too early to surround one's baby girl in the trappings that would "create a female aura round her." Pink accoutrements (from ribbons and ruffles to shoes, party dresses, and bracelets) symbolized the ideal vision of femininity. Pink think, as Peril describes it, has adapted to different generations and contexts.

Children's television programming frequently uses pink think to begin the gender socialization process, and children who watch the most television tend to hold the most stereotypic, gender-typed values.[27] For example, the television show *The Power Puff Girls* (airing from 1998 to 2004) depicts the adventures of Blossom, Bubbles, and Buttercup. Capturing the inherent contradictions of femininity, the narrative from the first episode emphasizes the ideal that little girls ought to be nice, perfect, and good:

> Sugar, Spice and everything nice…These were the ingredients chosen to create the perfect little girls. But Professor Utonium accidentally added an extra ingredient to the concoction… CHEMICAL X! Thus the Power Puff girls were born! And using their ultra super powers, Blossom, Bubbles and Buttercup have dedicated their lives to fighting crime and the forces of EVIL!!

CHEMICAL X in the story line alludes to the female sex chromosomes. Instead of adding a Y to the base chromosomal pair to make little boys, the creator made a mistake and accidentally added an X, creating the XX combination. The little girls were born. This story line neatly establishes the binary gender classification system for its young viewers. The inadvertent creation of the girls suggests male sex preference, and the devaluation of the feminine. Once a binary system is in place, the traits associated with the feminine take their official place within it. The little girls' softness (puff) offsets their power and suggests malleability, while their lifetime of dedication to fighting crime and evil indicates selflessness and high moral fortitude.

In contrast, the *Batman* epic on television, movies, and comic books provides a masculine counterpoint to the femininity embedded in the *Power Puff Girls*. The classic story of Batman reveals an underlying masculine ideology that is tied to male violence, punishment, and instant justice.[28] These characteristics are a deliberate response to intense anger. For Batman, his anger stems from a childhood trauma in which he witnessed the death of his parents. In avenging their deaths, Batman holds high moral standing in an ancient battle of good against evil. Although the *Girls* also fight evil from a moral standpoint, their motivations and attitudes correspond with gender-specific stereotypes that equate girls and women with the emotions of happiness, sadness, and fear; on the contrary, anger is associated with men.[29] Especially when calculated, men's public displays of anger reinforce the binary gender system. The contrasting characteristics of aggressive/passive, rational/emotional, hardness/softness, and seriousness/frivolity set Batman and the *Girls* apart as super heroes/she-roes.

Since gender socialization continues throughout a person's life, gender stereotypes find receptive audiences throughout the cultural marketplace. Pink femininity has become an especially fashionable commodity. Heir to the Hilton hotel fortune, Paris Hilton represents the popular face of pink femininity for teens and young women. In addition to claiming pink as her favorite color, Hilton presents herself as femininity in modern form, readily exhibiting her "pink tech"—hip cell phones, MP3 players, digital cameras, and other pink devices. The media attention she receives from tabloid and official news sources also upholds Ms. Hilton as an embodiment of femininity. In her pink-covered book *Confessions of an Heiress,* Hilton illustrates the feminine ideal:[30]

> If you act like a doormat, no one will lift a finger for you. This does not mean you should *ever* be mean, or snobby. A true heiress is never mean to anyone—except a girl who steals her boyfriend. An heiress should be a little above it all, but sweet… And she shouldn't go around spilling her guts to everyone. Have some secrets, I say. Secrets are very important assets if you are going to be an heiress.

Hilton considers herself to be a role model for young women, and she outlines the rules of pink femininity: be sweet, but not a doormat; be superior, but reserved and secretive.

Similar to the earlier visions of femininity, sweetness mitigates power and there are few situations that warrant overt expressions of anger. Within a melodramatic narrative, Hilton's portrayal reinforces social expectations that women should exhibit a pink façade that includes a feminine appearance, conciliatory behavior, emotional sensitivity, social restraint, and, of course, pink accessories.

Pink Femininity in Breast Cancer Culture

The culture of breast cancer draws on the institutional strength of the existing gender system and incorporates pink femininity into its symbols, messages, and stories to feminize breast cancer. The use of the color pink in the breast cancer ribbon easily conjures the imagery and discourse of pink femininity. The cultural representations in pink ribbon culture include national, regional, and local advertising campaigns and promotional materials, cause-marketing advertisements, newspaper and television stories, popular reference and self-help books, published breast cancer biographies, Internet sites and blogs, plot lines in movies and television shows, organizational newsletters, and press releases. These resources are self-referential and mutually reinforcing, forming a narrative structure that incorporates aspects of pink femininity, thereby feminizing pink ribbon culture. Abundant throughout mass media, these representations ensure the mass distribution of the culture they produce and serve as explicit guides about how to be an exemplary breast cancer survivor or supporter.

Beyond the high incidence of breast cancer among women, breast cancer's association with pink femininity helps to femi-nize it, or define it as a woman's illness. Focusing on goodness, morality, and women's domain in the family/private sphere, the pink ribbon evokes feminine purity and virtue. Barbara Katz Rothman writes: "Breast cancer is the disease of innocence, of mothers, grandmothers, aunts, and sisters. It is a disease that grows at home, not out there in dirty places."[31] The breast can-cer movement strategically and successfully used this message to maintain the image of breast cancer as a good and important cause.[32] Persuading individuals and organizations to act on its behalf as a women's health epidemic, the fight against breast cancer positioned women themselves to take action in the war against breast cancer from a moral standpoint. At the same time, the discourse of pink femininity conveys the culturally accept-able ways for women to do so.

The personal story—in articles, books, advertisements, or sound bites—draws on the one-dimensional, character-driven focus of the melodramatic genre to convey the simple message that breast cancer is a source for women's personal transforma-tion. As is common in the melodramatic genre, stories center on emotional excess and women's place in the social world. In pink ribbon culture, these stories feature the emotions of pink femininity—happiness, sadness, and fear. I picked up *Smiling Thru the Tears: A Breast Cancer Survivor Odyssey* at a breast cancer awareness conference where the author, Pamela deLeon-Lewis, was a key-note speaker. The self-published collection of the author's poems conveys an epic journey with breast cancer. By characterizing her experience as an odyssey, the collection conjures dramatic, archetypal imagery full of good and evil, challenge and triumph. The title and introduction of *Smiling Thru* positions women's emotionality at the center of the breast cancer experience. The author describes an "emotional roller coaster on which [her] feelings, physical health, faith, and convictions were riding during this very stressful and life-changing phase of [her] life."[33]

Happiness is the emotion that prevails in this story, confirming the importance of sanguinity for the breast cancer survivor. In the poem "Most of the Times," the author describes the excessive emotionality that left her frustrated, but later transformed: "Sometimes I really lost it…I would succumb to the pressures around me. On my emotions I would take a ride. I'd fuss, I'd cuss, I'd cry in frustration until there was nothing left inside."[34] Her dramatic expression of sadness and the fear that is associated with wishing one's reality were different is replaced with an optimistic solution only three lines later: "But I know, now, those days were really needed. I had to vent and set myself free." In the breast cancer drama that dominates pink ribbon culture, the story line is one of emotional upheaval, ultimately ending in triumph and happiness.

The heightened value of optimism is also a gender-consistent emotional expression for women in the broader culture.[35] The author of *Cancer Vixen*, Marisa Acocella Marchetto, confirms in an interview with Random House the importance of a positive attitude. In the quotation that opens this chapter,

Marchetto does not say that her cancer is in remission, but that her "negativity" is. Later in the interview, she states: "In many ways, believe it or not, I look at the whole experience as something positive. It made me a better person, a better wife, a better daughter, a better stepmother, a better sister, a better friend, and ultimately led me to a better life."[36] Marchetto repeats the word "better" seven times. Unlike Lance Armstrong's use of aggrandizing words described previously to present himself as dominant, Marchetto's use of these words suggests that she was not good enough prior to her breast cancer experience. Importantly, Marchetto's litany of improvements involves her social roles, stressing the relational orientation prevalent in the feminine ethos of cancer culture. By assigning a positive meaning to breast cancer and bearing witness to it through personal experience, the language and symbolism within the story help to produce a kind of reality about breast cancer, one that may or may not exist in *actual* reality. Yet, the continual retelling of the story establishes both a mode of survivorship and a model for the collective response to breast cancer.

Pink ribbon culture uses the transformational power of the personal story to convey dominant cultural scripts that construct a feminine illness identity. Almost all representations of breast cancer depict the same story of hope, courage, and joyous inspiration, stressing the importance of women's emotionality and relationships. "Breast cancer survivors describe how the disease has helped them salvage failing relationships, boost their self-confidence, establish new friendships, rethink their priorities, get in shape, and find true happiness."[37] *Chicken Soup for the Breast Cancer Survivor's Soul* features 101 stories to do the same. However, *Chicken Soup* exemplifies another prevalent pattern in the culture's construction of feminine illness identity: trivialization and infantilization.

The editor's book summary sends a light-hearted, inspirational message: "Going through the experience of breast cancer is no picnic, but with loving support, helpful advice and the healing power of laughter, it can be achieved." This opening sentence establishes a framework of informality, amusement, and a feminine care ethic as central to the breast cancer experience. These characteristics both feminize and devalue breast cancer. First, the idea of loving support suggests women's ethic of caring and the emotionality of the feminine. The feminine ethos of cancer culture calls upon women's nurturance, generosity, and inspiration to help other women. The excerpt later reiterates this point: "It is our fondest hope that you will be encouraged, buoyed, uplifted and instructed by the stories... Other breast-cancer survivors wrote them for you—to bring you hope, to give you strength and courage." A reciprocal care ethic goes a long way toward increasing social support. However, a well-developed literature on care work finds that gender structures care work in ways that put the primary responsibility on women and contributes to important differences in how women and men perceive and respond to illness.[38] Chapter 7 shows the complicated impact of women's responsibility for care work on those who are also facing breast cancer.

Second, the word *picnic* has never entered my mind as a way to describe breast cancer. Although the writer emphatically clarifies that breast cancer is *not* a picnic, the slang phraseology suggests informality and immediately trivializes the difficulty, fear, and pain that frequently accompanies breast cancer and treatment. While research has shown a general correlation between a positive attitude and well-being, the use of the word "laughter" reinforces the lack of seriousness. In the context of pink femininity, the feminine ethos of cancer culture, and the gender binary, the comedic portrayal of the tearful yet happy breast cancer survivor suggests immaturity and inadequacy.[39] Just as Marchetto's use of aggrandizing language suggested that she needed breast cancer to develop as a woman, pink ribbon culture (crowded with melodramatic personal stories and light-heartedness) reminds women that the problem of breast cancer can be solved if women know their place and do what they're told.

The zeal associated with pink is precisely because of its association with pink femininity. *Passionately Pink for the Cure*™ is a year-round fundraising/education program sponsored by Komen, in conjunction with National Breast Cancer Awareness Month. Komen's website states:

> More than the color for breast cancer awareness, pink represents the promise between <u>two sisters</u> to find a cure for breast cancer. That promise started the Komen Foundation and ignited the passion of millions to create a world without breast cancer. Are you passionate?

The association of pink with passion evokes femininity in terms of love, marriage, romance, sexuality, commitment, emotionality. These characteristics construct gender and identify proper social roles for women. When women are asked, "Are you passionate?" the answer must be a resounding YES if we are to keep our gender identities intact.

Following this example, a local breast health community outreach program sent an announcement to the faculty and staff at a local university to request survivor and co-survivor stories for Breast Cancer Awareness Month.

> Are you a breast cancer survivor, a co-survivor, or someone just passionately pink for the cause? If so, we'd love to hear from you! The [Outreach Program] is currently seeking survivor stories—messages that educate, empower, and encourage individuals to Think Pink! about early detection!...We invite you to lend your voice to raise awareness, offer support, and share compelling messages of strength, hope, and courage.

The norms and values of survivorship and support instill the message that there is a single way to speak about, and therefore experience, breast cancer. If a breast cancer survivor does not vehemently exhibit strength, hope, and courage, she is not *invited* to participate in pink ribbon culture. The culture demands public displays of she-roic values. Women's empowerment in this culture is defined in terms of women's compliance to its model of survivorship.

The She-ro

No model in pink ribbon culture captures the ethos of American cancer culture and pink femininity better than the *she-ro*. With feminine style, optimism, courage, humor, and resolve, this woman hero in pink fights breast cancer and wins. The she-ro represents an amalgamation of the masculine/feminine ethos, which enables her to garner social capital while accommodating the norms of pink femininity. Although the she-ro is a breast cancer survivor, she-roism is also open to women who have *not* been diagnosed with breast cancer. Presenting a united front in the war against breast cancer, the she-ro army walks, runs, and consumes in the name of the cause. The pink ribbon culture and its most powerful allies organize, fund, and publicize the she-ro army through an array of marketing strategies and public policy initiatives (Chapters 4 and 5). The norms and values of the culture, its imagery and discourse, stories and she-roes, come together to create an epic war on breast cancer. Although this war has been fought to some degree since the 1930s when the WFA enlisted, the modern war on breast cancer has a new arsenal, a larger army, and a more encompassing doctrine. The war is still fought in and through women's bodies, but it is also waged in the streets, on the airwaves, and in the identities of its soldiers and bystanders alike.

The she-ro is an ideal type, which embodies pink femininity and pink ribbon culture's model of survivorship. The primary purpose is to convey the norms and values of the culture to as many people as possible as often as possible, featuring the she-ro in personal stories, survivor profiles, announcements, posters, photos, and on products ad infinitum. She influences and transmits the culture of breast cancer while shaping individual and collective responses to the illness. There are many examples of the she-ro, even within the illustrations discussed in the previous section. A closer look at *Breast Cancer Odyssey*, for example, also reveals the adventures of a she-ro. In the midst of emotionality and personal transformation, the author depicts herself as "a born fighter" in a war she "must win," who "stands tall" proclaiming, "Kiss my butt, Cancer!"[40] With humor, war rhetoric, and a smile, the she-ro's story is the one that gets representation in pink ribbon culture.

The quintessential example of she-ro is *Cancer Vixen*.[41] With a superhero feel reminiscent of the *Power Puff Girls,* the author-protagonist of this graphic memoir about her breast cancer experience is the she-ro of the story. Like deLeon-Lewis, Cancer Vixen also proclaims, "Cancer, I am gonna kick your butt."[42] Embodying the paradoxes of the masculine/feminine ethos, she adds: "And, I'm gonna do it in killer five-inch heels."[43] The illustration on the front cover depicts the drama of a slender young woman with long, blonde hair. Wearing a mini-skirt and open-toed high heels that reveal her pink toenails, the Vixen demonstrates a high martial arts kick.

Cancer Vixen displays pink femininity while taking on masculine power and aggression. She is emotional, sexually attractive, and tough, and the combination of these characteristics confers social status: after all she is a vixen, not a victim. Drawing attention to her survivor status and sexual acumen, *Cancer Vixen* exemplifies Maren Klawiter's observation that "unlike the victim of yesteryear, [the new breast cancer survivor] was a woman whose femininity, sexuality and desirability were intact." Regardless of reconstruction, prosthetics, and reproductive potential, pink femininity provides an aesthetic solution to the disruption of breast cancer.

Ellen Leopold argues that the evolution of attitudes toward breast cancer from being taboo to becoming part of almost every cultural medium required a shift in representation.[44]

Pink attitude and accoutrements were the catalyst to change the face of breast cancer. Now, feminine style and good cheer are the most important aspects of the she-ro's victory over the disease. Upbeat stories like *Cancer Vixen* use a melodramatic tone to successfully convey she-roism. The Vixen plot line:

> She argues with her mother (whom she dubs "smother"); cries an ocean of tears with a gaggle of best friends; questions God ("Hey you up there, how could you make me a bald, unhealthy, baggage-ridden bride?"); marries her long-time love; and dabbles in cabala. She also makes a point of wearing designer shoes to her chemo sessions. Session 2: Giuseppe Zanotti sandals. Session 6: White patent leather pumps by Hotel Venus.[45]

Soap operas, television dramas, movies, and comedies integrate health issues to enrich plots, and sometimes convey health information.[46] The Vixen's dramatic, emotional, and funny story echoes a plotline in the dramatic comedy *Sex and the City* in which one of the leading characters, Samantha, was diagnosed with breast cancer after seeking breast enlargement. Samantha's breast cancer experience makes its way into several episodes to reiterate the emotional excess, chaos, and feminine accessories involved in the she-ro's eventual triumph.

While humor and light-heartedness can be used to express and negotiate the tensions of breast cancer and convey informational messages, the telling and retelling of the she-ro story in and beyond the culture do something else. They concretize the rules of engagement for any woman who is diagnosed with, or at risk for, breast cancer. They trivialize breast cancer by presenting it with a comedic and melodramatic tenor. Entertainment and melodrama are the most degraded and devalued of genres.[47] The personal stories often use this genre or its qualities to make breast cancer palatable for public consumption, and it works. *Glamour's* editor-in-chief said about *Cancer Vixen*: "We liked that it was light and funny and she wasn't being too reverent...You couldn't hear the violins in the background playing."[48] Similarly, Kris Carr's book *Crazy Sexy Cancer Tips*, based on her personal experience with cancer, is laugh-out-loud funny and has an entire chapter on "retail therapy."[49] CBS News correspondent Kelly Wallace says it may be "the first girlfriend's guide to living with cancer."[50]

Pink ribbon culture accommodates generational differences between the "personal is political" sentiment of second-wave feminism and the use of commercial and popular culture as forms of resistance within feminism's third wave.[51] As discussed in Chapter 2, the breast cancer movement focused on the centrality of women's experiences as breast cancer survivors, educators, and informed decision-makers who could influence collective action, public policy, and their own health. At the same time, the culture that grew out of women's organizing integrated elements of third-wave feminism, which defines women's empowerment in terms of commercial media visibility and the symbolic power that comes with it. The she-ro is part of a general trajectory in contemporary mass media that can, in part, be attributed to the "girl power" of third-wave feminism. The she-ro is a power puff girl who grew up and got breast cancer. Playing on generational differences between the second and third feminist waves, pink ribbon culture declares women's empowerment through the use of she-roism, a homogenized version of women's advocacy coupled with mass-mediated consumption.

The new war on breast cancer is an epic war—a massively supported, well-funded, mass-mediated war of representation and identity. With deep ties to corporate sponsorship, anyone can be a warrior for the cause. She-roism is no longer the exclusive domain of the breast cancer survivor.

NOTES

1. Random House, Inc. Interview with Marisa Acocella Marchetto. Random House.http://www.randomhouse.com/catalog/display.pperl?isbn=9780307263575&view=auqa.

2. B. Lerner, *The Cancer Wars: Hope, Fear, and the Pursuit of a Cure in Twentieth-Century America* (New York: Oxford University Press, 2001), 44.

3. E. Leopold, *A Darker Ribbon: Breast Cancer, Women, and Their Doctors in the Twentieth Century* (Boston: Beacon Press, 1999), 12-13.

4. Lerner, *The Cancer Wars*.

5. F. S. Slaughter, *The New Science of Surgery* (New York: Julian Messner, 1946), 244. Quoted in Lerner, *The Cancer Wars*, 60.

6. Mary Douglas, *Purity and Danger: An Analysis of Concepts of Pollution and Taboo* (1966; repr., New York: Routledge, 1984). Douglas argues that ambiguity is a source of powerful symbolism within cultures because societies tend to view ambiguous phenomena as dangerous. Thus, to deal with ambiguity, first the phenomenon is socially assigned to one of two possible categories (i.e., normal/abnormal, good/bad, health/illness, masculine/feminine, pure/polluted, and so on). Then, it is avoided whenever possible. Or, if an anomalous situation materializes that cannot be categorized or avoided, it is destroyed. In the gender order, the feminine side of the binary classification parallels the abnormal, bad, ill, polluted. Thus, femininity itself comprises its own set of conflicting classifications.

7. C. West & D. Zimmerman, "Doing Gender," *Gender and Society* 1 (1987): 125-51.

8. R. Descartes, "Meditations on First Philosophy," in *The Philosophical Writings of Descartes*, vol. 2, trans. J. Cottingham, R. Stoothoff & D. Murdoch (Cambridge: Cambridge University Press, 1984).

9. Susan Sontag, *Illness as Metaphor and AIDS and Its Metaphors* (New York: Picador, 2001); C. Seale, "Sporting Cancer: Struggle Language in News Reports of People with Cancer," Sociology of Health and Illness 23 no. 3 (2001): 308-29.

10. About Us: Milestones. LIVE**STRONG** Lance Armstrong Foundation. http://www.livestrong.org/site/c.khLXK1PxHmF/b.2662471/k.26F8/Milestones.htm; FAQs. Gilda's Club Worldwide. http://www.

gildasclub.org/faqs.asp. G. Radner, *It's Always Something*. (New York: Harper Entertainment, 2000).

11. R. W. Connell, *Gender and Power* (Stanford, CA: Stanford University Press, 1987).

12. About Us: Lance's Story. LIVE**STRONG** Lance Armstrong Foundation. http://www.livestrong.org/site/c.khLXK1PxHmF/b.2661053/k.9207/Lances_Story.htm.

13. R. Murphy, *The Body Silent: The Different World of the Disabled* (New York: W. W. Norton, 2001).

14. Livestrong Presidential Cancer Forum. http://www.kintera.org/AutoGen/ecard/cardForm.asp?ievent=245271.

15. Sontag, *Illness as Metaphor*.

16. Lance Armstrong & Sally Jenkins, *It's Not About the Bike: My Journey Back to Life* (New York: Putnam, 2000); Lance Armstrong, with Sally Jenkins, *Every Second Counts* (New York: Broadway Books, 2003).

17. About Us: Financial Information. Financial Statements. 2006 and 2005 audited combined financial statements. http://www.livestrong.org/site/c.khLXK1PxHmF/b.2662367/k.5D4A/Financial_Information.htm.

18. S. Jenkins, "Let's Get to Work," *The Washington Post*, September 10, 2008, E01.

19. J. Hockenberry, *Moving Violations: War Zones, Wheelchairs, and Declarations of Independence* (New York: Hyperion, 1995); J. Lorber & L. J. Moore, *Gender and the Social Construction of Illness* (Lanham, MD: Rowman & Littlefield, 2002).

20. Men of the Week: Sports. Askmen.com. http://www.askmen.com/men/sports/40_lance_armstrong.html.

21. FAQs. Gilda's Club Worldwide.

22. Gilda's Legacy. Gilda's Club Worldwide. http://www.gildasclub.org/faqs.asp.

23. Gilda's Club Language. Gilda's Club Worldwide. http://www.gildasclub.org/philosophy.asp.

24. Advocacy Role. Gilda's Club Worldwide. http://www.gildasclub.org/ourorganization.asp.

25. Radner, *It's Always Something*.

26. L. Peril, *Pink Think: Becoming a Woman in Many Uneasy Lessons* (New York: W. W. Norton & Company, 2002).

27. Mark Barner, "Sex-Role Stereotyping In FCC-Mandated Children's Educational Television," *Journal of Broadcasting and Electronic Media* 43, no. 4 (Fall 1999): 551-64; Stacy L. Smith & Barbara J. Wilson, "Television Viewing, Fat Stereotyping, Body Shape Standards, and Eating Disorder Symptomatology in Grade School Children," *Communication Research* 27, no. 5 (2000): 617-41; D. Birnbaum, "Preschoolers' Stereotypes About Sex Differences In Emotionality: A Reaffirmation," *Journal of Genetic Psychology,* 143 (1983): 139-40.

28. G. Newman, "Batman and Justice: The True Story," *Humanity and Society* 17, no. 3 (1993): 297-320.

29. D. Birnbaum, T. Nosanchuk, & W. Croll, "Children's Stereotypes about Sex Differences in Emotionality," *Sex Roles* 6 (1980): 435-43; N. Briton & J. Hall, "Beliefs About Female and Male Nonverbal Communication," *Sex Roles* 32 (1995): 79-90; R. Fabes & C. Martin, "Gender and Age Stereotypes of Emotionality," *Personality and Social Psychology Bulletin* 17 (1991): 532-40; M. Grossman & W. Wood, "Sex Differences in Intensity of Emotional Experience: A Social Role Interpretation," *Journal of Personality and Social Psychology* 65 (1993): 1010-22; J. R. Kelly & S. L. Hutson-Comeaux, "Gender-Emotion Stereotypes Are Context Specific," *Sex Roles* 40 (1999): 107-20.

30. P. Hilton, M. Ginsberg, & J. Vespa, *Confessions of an Heiress: A Tongue-in-Chic Peek Behind the Pose* (New York: Simon & Schuster, 2004), 5.

31. B. K. Rothman, "Genetic Technology and Women," in *Women, Gender, and Technology,* ed. M. F. Fox, D. G. Johnson, & S. V. Rosser, 118 (Urbana: University of Illnois Press, 2006).

32. B. Brenner, "Sister Support," in *Breast Cancer: Society Shapes an Epidemic*, ed. A. Kasper & S. Ferguson, 328-9 (New York: Palgrave 2000); M. Klawiter, "Breast Cancer in Two Regimes: The Impact of Social Movements on Illness Experience," *Sociology of Health and Illness* 26 (September 2004): 845-74; Klawiter, "From Private Stigma to Global Assembly"; C. Seale, "Sporting Cancer."

33. P. DeLeon-Lewis, *Smiling Thru the Tears: A Breast Cancer Survivor Odyssey* (Baltimore: Publish America, 2005), 7.

34. *Ibid.*, 135.

35. C. G. Geerand & S. A. Shields, "Women and Emotion: Stereotypes and the Double Bind," in *Lectures on the Psychology of Women*, ed. J. C. Chrisler, C. Golden, & P. D. Rozee, 63-73 (New York: McGraw-Hill, 1996).

36. Random House, Inc. Interview with Marisa Acocella Marchetto.

37. King, *Pink Ribbons Inc.*, 102.

38. E. K. Abel & M. K. Nelson, *Circles of Care* (Albany: SUNY Press, 1990); J. Aronson, "Sense of Responsibility for the Care of Old People: 'But Who Else Is Going to Do It?'" *Gender and Society* 6, no. 1 (1992): 8-29; M. Duffy, "Reproducing Labor Inequalities: Challenges for Feminists Conceptualizing Care at the Intersections of Gender, Race, and Class," *Gender and Society* 19, no. 1 (2005): 66-82; N. Gerstel & S. Gallagher, "Men's Caregiving: Gender and the Contingent Character of Care," *Gender and Society* 15, no. 2 (2001): 197-217; P. Herd & M. Harrington Meyer, "Care Work: Invisible Civic Engagement," *Gender and Society* 16, no. 5 (2002): 665-88.

39. B. Ehrenreich, "Welcome to Cancerland: A Mammogram Leads to a Cult of Pink Kitsch," *Harper's Magazine* (Nov. 2001): 43-53. Ehrenreich explains the infantilizing trope of the breast cancer marketplace: "in some versions of the prevailing gender ideology, femininity is by its nature incompatible with full adulthood—a state of arrested development."

40. DeLeon-Lewis, *Smiling Thru the Tears*, 27, 33, 51.

41. Random House, Inc. Interview with Marisa Acocella Marchetto.

42. *Ibid.*

43. *Ibid.*

44. King, *Pink Ribbons, Inc.*; Klawiter, *Breast Cancer in Two Regimes*; Leopold, *A Darker Ribbon*; E. S. Kolker, "Framing as a Cultural Resource in Health Social Movements: Funding Activism and the Breast Cancer Movement in the US, 1990–1993," *Sociology of Health and Illness* 266 (2004): 820-44.

45. L. Ogunnaike, "A Vixen Cartooning in the Face of Cancer," *The New York Times,* April 14, 2005. http://www.nytimes.com/2005/04/14/books/14canc.html?_r=1&ex=1187582400&en=00885b4bc94ee063&ei=5070.

46. M. Brodie, U. Foehr, V. Rideout, N. Baer, et al., "Communicating Health Information Through the Entertainment Media," *Health Affairs* 20 (2001): 192-200; A. Howe, V. Owen-Smith, & J. Richardson, "The Impact of a Television Soap Opera on the NHS Cervical Screening Programme in the North West of England," *Journal of Public Health Medicine* 24, no. 4 (2002): 299-304.

47. R. Jacobs & G. Sulik, "Ethnic and Gender Stereotypes in the Media," in *Encyclopedia of International Media and Communications,* ed. D. Johnston, 587-96. (San Diego: Academic Press, 2003).

48. Ogunnaike, "A Vixen Cartooning."

49. K. Carr, *Crazy Sexy Cancer Tips* (Guilford, CT: skirt! 2007).

50. *Crazy Sexy Cancer Tips*: Editorial Reviews. Amazon.com. http://www.amazon.com/Crazy-Sexy-Cancer-Tips-Kris/dp/B0019MU66G/ref=pd_sim_b_1.

51. C. Driscoll, Girls: Feminine Adolescence in Popular Culture and Cultural History (New York: Columbia University Press, 2002).

FOUR

CONSUMING PINK

Mass Media and the Conscientious Consumer

If you're a woman, you're at risk for breast cancer. Until there is a cure or ways to prevent the disease, one of the most important things you can do is get screened regularly. Help us spread the message by joining our Race to keep hope alive.

MAGAZINE ADVERTISEMENT: THE SUSAN G. KOMEN
BREAST CANCER FOUNDATION RACE FOR THE
CURE. ©2006. THE SUSAN G. KOMEN BREAST
CANCER FOUNDATION

I n a modern capitalist society, everything has its price—food, clothing, shelter, education, healthcare, information, ideas, and even advocacy. Marketing and advertising are pervasive, and those who sell Americans our way of life use these promotional strategies to influence how we spend our money. The culture that arises from consumption-based logic shapes what we believe to be important and worthwhile, what we do in everyday life, and how we do it. Likewise, a culture of consumption influences Americans' understanding of, and social responses to, social issues of the day. Breast cancer is no different. An advertisement in a popular women's magazine for the Komen Race for the Cure states unequivocally that women are at risk for breast cancer and that screening is of utmost importance. The ad directs women to spread this message by registering (paying a fee) for a Komen event, which involves soliciting pledges to raise funds for the organization in the name of breast cancer.

The marketing of breast cancer is associated with the consumption of information, medicine, technology, social support, events, food, paraphernalia—and an audience for all of these products and services. The audience of breast cancer survivors, women at risk, and supporters is the most highly valued product in the political economy of breast cancer, and corporations within and beyond the breast cancer industry pay large sums of money for access. In 1996, Lisa Belkin wrote that breast cancer had become the "darling of corporate America." Samantha King's analysis of the political economy of breast cancer in *Pink Ribbons, Inc.* explains that corporations, politicians, and consumers alike use the purchase of breast cancer-related goods and services as a proxy for good will and responsible citizenship.[2] As earlier chapters demonstrate, the packaging of breast cancer in terms of pink femininity, the broader cancer culture, and the history of the breast cancer movement has solidified breast cancer's social status and cultural accessibility. Breast cancer is indeed the darling of corporations—but it also has the power of celebrity, symbolism, myth, and the attention of mass media.

Without mass media as the primary vehicle for the dissemination of breast cancer culture, breast cancer would *not* have achieved the notoriety necessary to dominate the public imagination or the brand portfolios of major corporations. The culture surrounding breast cancer thrives in the mass-mediated world of representation. A pink ribbon culture provides the cultural platform and discursive framework through which mass media and consumption operate both as tools for the culture and as driving forces in their own right. As a result, breast cancer has become one of the most mass-mediated illnesses of our time.

THE SPECIAL ROLE OF
WOMEN'S MAGAZINES

Breast cancer news items, health updates, human interest stories, public service campaigns, community events, biographies, entertainment, and advertisements saturate the American media. Given that breast cancer was closeted into the 1960s, this transformation is remarkable. Women's magazines have been a vital part of breast cancer's entrée into mass culture. Historically, women's magazines/journals have been important for women as a group, creating a *virtual community* in which women who were relegated to the private sphere of home and hearth could access the public sphere of famous writers, political figures, and agitators for social justice. Targeting an upper-class female audience, the journals emphasized gender-appropriate topics such as fashion, culture, and fine arts. They also included fiction, self-help articles, and guides related to "women's work." Magazines are convenient, easy to pick up and put down, and are an inexpensive form of leisure. If the medical establishment wanted to spread its messages about breast cancer to women, women's magazines would be a good place to start.

Mary Ellen Zuckerman's *History of Popular Women's Magazines in the United States*[3] traces the successful development of women's magazines as an important new media form. A collection known as "The Big Six" included *Delineator, McCall's, Ladies' Home Journal, Woman's Home Companion, Good Housekeeping*, and *Pictorial Review*. The Big Six went on to top circulation in the first half of the 20th century, attracted considerable advertising dollars, and had thousands of loyal women readers. In 1937 *Delineator* merged into *Pictorial Review*, which stopped publication 2 years later. However, the remaining women's magazines continued to gain prominence, and breast cancer's increasing presence within them reflected the growing social importance of this illness to American society.

Accompanying basic breast cancer information, women's magazines supplied cultural messages. Themes pertained to women's role in the doctor–patient relationship, the personal characteristics thought to bring women what they needed to cope with breast cancer, war metaphor, traditional femininity, and the positioning of breast cancer as a major threat to women physically and socially. In May 1947, *Ladies' Home Journal* published an article that conjured the image of the omnipotent doctor, as patient Marion Flexner "tried hard not to disappoint" her physician husband when he told her she would need a mastectomy if her breast lump was cancerous.[4] Later that year, the magazine published a story about Mary Roberts Rinehart's experience, emphasizing how her diligent action was crucial for "beat[ing] her biggest opponent."[5] In accord with women's roles in society, women's action on behalf of their health was defined in terms of compliance to medical protocols and dependence on men, both husbands and doctors.

The push to normalize breast cancer screening as a regular part of healthy women's lives is a common form of medicalization—when medical definitions, diagnostics, and interventions spread into the normal, everyday lives of people. Women's magazines throughout the 1950s packaged medicalizing processes in ways that incorporated traditional gender expectations for sociability, feminine etiquette, and women's place in society. A 1955 *Good Housekeeping* article reported that over 5 million women had attended screenings of a film on "Breast Self-Examination" released by the American Cancer Society and the National Cancer Institute.[6] The article could have been titled, "Come On, Everybody's Doing It!" The organizations sponsoring the film and the magazine used an entertainment genre and popularity to convince women that screening was a good idea. The medicalization process—from diagnosis to treatment—simultaneously focused on women's dependence on men and patriarchal medicine.

Woman's Home Companion (1955) provided detailed information about post-diagnostic procedures, as a cancer expert outlined the hospital stay, anesthetic processes, biopsy and mastectomy procedures, and scarring. The article even discussed potential psychological aspects of mastectomy: "If you are married, you may worry that your husband will not accept your "mutilated" state. If you are single you may envision yourself no longer able to compete with other women for a husband."[7] These articles were published at the same time gynecology was developing as a surgical specialty and gynecologists considered a wide range of women's complaints to be the psychogenic result of women's rejection of femininity.[8]

To this point in the history of medicine, medical men (particularly surgeons) held unquestioned authority. In addition to dictating treatments and recommendations, doctors decided whether or not to tell women *the truth* about their diagnoses and prognoses.[9] A survey of doctors' attitudes in 1961 found that 90 percent of those who responded said they would regularly withhold the truth from their patients, even though there was evidence that women wanted to know the truth. Expressing this sentiment, *Ladies' Home Journal* published an article in 1961 with the provocative title: "Should Doctors Tell the Truth to a Cancer Patient?" The article reported that two thirds of women in a national survey from the Canadian Cancer Society said "yes." Still, women in the United States were not in a position to press for the truth. Indeed, that was a key rallying point of the women's health movement of the 1970s that focused on empowerment and the elevation of women's status as patients. However, most stories in women's magazines reflected a bias toward medical authority and the opinion of the expert long after the women's health movement succeeded in making significant changes.

From 1913 to 1996, there were more than 250 articles (averaging three per year) about breast cancer in 11 of the most popular women's magazines in the United States. The majority of these articles (70 percent) were written in the voice of the expert. Coupled with messages of personal responsibility to encourage specific behaviors, the stories valorized medical opinion and authority. *Ladies' Home Journal* stated that their 1969 guide to breast self-examination was "intended to help you know more about your breasts, but not to help you make judgments about your health. Leave that to your doctor."[10] A 1996 *Good Housekeeping* article—nearly 30 years later—had the same message. The title "Courage that Runs in the Family" might lead the reader to believe that the article is about the personal attributes and perspectives of family members. Ultimately, however, the article reinforces the authority of the medical expert, presenting his opinion as truth: "Ruth Ann's doctor says the chemotherapy worked: her prognosis is good."[11] In an analysis of mass print media, Clarke finds that magazine articles such as this one assume that allopathic medicine and conventional medical treatment are the only appropriate responses to breast cancer.

Although personal accounts of breast cancer are now common, though largely contained to a narrow story line, women's magazines did not regularly share the voices of diagnosed women. The void in personal accounts became clear when celebrity Shirley Temple Black described her illness in *McCall's* in 1973. The month after her story, "Don't Sit Home and Be Afraid," was published, Black received over 50,000 letters. The magazine immediately printed a follow-up that described this correspondence as an "outpouring of love" for her courage in "rip[ping] away the veil of secrecy and shame" that surrounded breast cancer.[12] Black's notoriety drew attention to "the veil," but it had not really been lifted: the stigma associated with breast cancer remained strong despite the emergence of breast cancer organizations and the expansion of education and support programs. To enter the public realm fully, breast cancer needed the attention of media outlets that held greater social legitimacy.

Betty Ford's 1974 diagnosis extended the breast cancer discussion. Ford's political status as the first lady gave her experience public significance that piqued the interest of news media. Ford's statement in the November issue of *Time* magazine reveals that she was cognizant of her role: "The fact that I was the wife of the President put it in headlines and brought before the public this particular experience I was going through. It made a lot of women realize that it could happen to them. I'm sure I've saved at least one person—maybe more."[13] Then the article's focus shifted to another public figure, Happy Rockefeller, wife of Vice President-designate Nelson Rockefeller. After reading about Ford's well-publicized experience, the article states, Rockefeller decided to "do what doctors urge all women to do regularly: examine her breasts for suspicious growths... Happy's quick action may well have saved her life." The message of early detection, urgency, and the importance of medical intervention echoed the promotional campaigns from the American Cancer Society, as well as the stories about breast cancer in women's magazines. What was most significant about Ford and Rockefeller was that they had the political clout to elicit the kind of media attention that would raise breast cancer's legitimacy as a topic suitable for the general public.

The social legitimacy of breast cancer led to increased media interest. News stories tended to focus on basic information about cancer and its treatment, research on causes and prevention, and economic issues related to insurance and political issues,[14] but news media rarely focused on the social aspects of cancer such as personal survival or coping stories.[15] Women's magazines focused on basic information too, but they also concentrated on the personal perspective of the cancer patient. Similar to coverage of other illnesses, the majority of articles in the top women's magazines from 1913 to 1996 continued to be written in the voice of "the expert."

As the incidence of breast cancer continued to rise, its public presence grew, and breast cancer advocacy acquired greater national influence, women's magazines published a greater number of breast cancer-related stories.[16] By the mid-1990s breast cancer had become the most widely discussed cancer in women's magazines.[17] Ironically, these were the same magazines advertising cigarettes to women, now accounting for lung cancer deaths overtaking breast cancer in older women. Although the bulk of the articles continued to prioritize the voice of the expert, the perspective of the breast cancer survivor steadily gained prominence. A growing number of articles relied on quotes from diagnosed women, were written by women with breast cancer, or were personal narratives about women's experiences. By the end of the 20th century, breast cancer narratives were a genre of their own.[18]

THE BREAST CANCER AUDIENCE

For a social problem to dominate mass media, it must be socially important and culturally accessible to a clearly identifiable audience. Women's magazines historically catered to an upper-class group of women, thereby constructing a mainstream "women's audience" that integrated and (re)created class-based gender mores. In using women's magazines to reach women about breast cancer, the "women's audience" that these magazines targeted (and produced) inevitably shaped the contours of the "breast cancer audience." The rise of new technology in the 1970s dramatically expanded the number of mass media outlets, fracturing the audience and threatening the viability of women's magazines. In response, the magazines started to target specific niches, such as career women, feminists, and African American women. Fashion and lifestyle magazines in the 1980s offered cultural repertoires that catered to niche audiences. They also provided practical information about how to live a particular type of lifestyle. For women, this involved advice on relationships and men, as well as topical features related to beauty, fashion, career, and the latest news about health topics such as breast cancer.

In a mass-mediated consumer culture, the niche audience is a highly valued commodity.[19] Companies and organizations use a variety of strategies to reach niche audiences, with the goal of influencing behavior and consumption. In reaching audiences through word of mouth, advertising, interactions with a company or its representatives, and real-life experiences, companies and organizations produce and reinforce audience composition. A magazine may advertise a product (e.g., stylish shoes) that targets active career women in their thirties. The same magazine references a popular movie (e.g., *Sex and the City*), which also targets this group. When career women in their thirties read the magazine, watch the movie, discuss the characters at work, or buy the product, they become associated with the characteristics of the niche audience and reinforce its boundaries. If the movie was based on the television show (which had an episode about breast cancer), the magazine has a story about breast cancer, and the shoe advertisement states that the company gives a portion of sales to breast cancer research; then, the audience of "career women in their thirties" becomes associated with breast cancer. This is one of the ways the breast cancer audience is produced. However, the breast cancer audience is larger and broader than this singular niche.

Pink ribbon culture plays a key role in defining the breast cancer audience. Breast cancer organizations market personal experiences, empowerment rhetoric, and social networks to increase publicity while raising funds. Real-life experiences and word of mouth increase social awareness of breast cancer as an important problem and disseminate cultural repertoires about how to deal with the illness. Organizations and companies advertise these same repertoires while selling their products and services. Individuals who consume these products and services become part of the audience and use their personal experiences to lend legitimacy to the cause. These strategies produce a breast cancer audience that goes beyond breast cancer survivors to include women at risk and a general category of supporters.

The *survivor* represents the primary niche in the breast cancer audience. As discussed in Chapter 3, representations in pink ribbon culture highlight the status of the survivor by encouraging identification with the she-ro as an embodiment of the masculine (courage and victorious resolve) and the feminine (light-hearted optimism and panache). Personal stories and copious accounts of the she-ro experience reverberate throughout breast cancer organizing and activities. Although the she-ro represents the ultimate breast cancer survivor, the qualities of the she-ro (she-roism) can be applied to *women at risk* and a multitude of *supporters* of the cause. Experts in pink ribbon culture report that "being a woman" is the primary risk factor for developing breast cancer, which means that all women are at risk.[20] The implication is that *all* women are part of the breast cancer audience. Sustained and increasing incidence rates provide evidence that women's risk is high, and the heightened visibility of survivors impels people to reveal their survivor status openly, thereby providing even more evidence of women's risk. Though some keep their diagnoses hidden, the contemporary cultural environment encourages disclosure. Heightened anxiety about women's risk and personal knowledge about diagnosed family members, friends, and acquaintances encourage the public to think about breast cancer—thereby creating the third niche of supporters.

"Warrior? Survivor? Supporter? Which One Are You?" This slogan is from a poster for a 2007 community breast cancer walk. The purpose of the event is to raise money for the sponsoring organization, whose mission is to provide funding for local breast cancer outreach and support services. This purpose harks back to one of the early goals of the breast cancer movement: to provide material and emotional support to breast cancer survivors. Such history lends legitimacy to the event and to the organization's purpose. The event slogan then draws on pink ribbon culture to delineate three roles one can play as a member of the breast cancer audience: warrior, survivor, or supporter. In asking the public which role defines them, the message is that at least one of them should. Since the warrior is the first option, it is the preferred role. In pink ribbon culture the she-ro is the ultimate survivor-warrior. However, in contemporary mass media and other cultural representations of breast cancer, as I will discuss later in this chapter, anyone can be a supporter-warrior for the cause.

Two media events were crucial in expanding the breast cancer audience beyond the survivor role: (1) the 1985 televised kickoff of National Breast Cancer Awareness Month (NBCAM) and (2) the 1992 debut of the pink ribbon. Pharmaceutical giant AstraZeneca established NBCAM as a campaign to capitalize on women's desire to know "the truth" about breast cancer, and Betty Ford and her daughter agreed to be spokespersons. Claiming to "fill the information void," NBCAM's mission was to educate and empower women to "take charge of their own breast health." The program defines this undertaking as "practicing regular self-breast exams...scheduling regular visits and annual mammograms with their healthcare provider, adhering to prescribed treatment, and knowing the facts about recurrence."[21] Although it started as a week-long event, NBCAM became a year-long series of educational and fundraising activities culminating in October. NBCAM consists of "the creation and distribution of promotional materials, brochures, advertisements, public service spots, and other educational aids." In addition to advertising, NBCAM obtains free exposure through word of mouth, clinical promotion, workplace and community initiatives, and political representatives. In promoting regular surveillance and screening for breast cancer survivors and undiagnosed women, NBCAM concretizes the niche audience of women at risk.

The official unveiling of the pink ribbon in 1992 furthered the NBCAM agenda and solidified the place of breast cancer in public relations, marketing, and mass media. As the symbol for breast cancer awareness, the pink ribbon provided a new strategy for maintaining public interest in breast cancer and disseminating the message of early detection. Once again, women's magazines played a vital role. In 1991 *Self* magazine had already dedicated an issue to NBCAM, with guest editor Evelyn Lauder. NBCAM continues to use the pink ribbon to foster a specific association between breast cancer awareness and early detection. However, NBCAM and a variety of organizations and companies also use the symbol to create a general sense of awareness, to raise funds, and to affiliate with the cause. Within a discursive framework that integrates the broader cancer culture with the empowerment rhetoric, gender norms, and marketing strategies of pink ribbon culture, the pink ribbon helps to affirm the breast cancer audience, increase media attention, and market a *breast cancer brand*.

BRANDING AND THE NICHE MARKET OF THE SOCIALLY AWARE

Symbolic expressions of information, experiences, identities, and associations construct audiences and produce cultural repertoires for them to use in interpreting the world around them. Cultural representations (including advertisements, promotional materials, and mass media) are a dimension of social reality in which people learn what should frighten them, offer them hope, and make them feel good about themselves and their situations. As an agent for the transmission of pink femininity and cancer culture, pink ribbon symbolism is accessible and translates well to mass-mediated cultural forms. It is the friendly, optimistic, attractive, and unequivocal aspects of pink ribbon culture that forge a lasting relationship between the cause of breast cancer and the breast cancer audience. This relationship enforces the principal message that breast cancer is an important cause, and that supporting it indicates good will toward women. This message is so strong and consistent across cultural representations in pink ribbon culture that breast cancer now functions as a brand, with a pink ribbon logo. Analyzing breast cancer as a brand sheds light on the use of this illness in advertising and promotional campaigns that encourage consumption in the name of the cause.

Branding is geared toward influencing long-term consumption practices, loyalty, and cultural identity. As exemplary forms of media imagery, brands can be used to construct niche markets and influence the character of the consumer audience. To guarantee loyalty, many companies create brands that represent an attitude or feeling that is based on the perceived needs of the consumer. Many brands are designed to influence how consumers think of themselves. For instance, Nike's slogan "Just Do It" dares consumers to take action and challenge themselves to achieve something, anything. In the context of sports and Nike's athletic endorsements, the message encourages individuals to engage in physical activity that likely requires Nike's athletic shoes. However, the brand need not be connected to a product at all. Nike tapped into an important American belief oriented to hard work and getting ahead. Igniting a purpose beyond the mere purchase of Nike's products, the brand fosters a *cultural identity* that resonates with the audience.

The branding of ideas, attitudes, and social issues is now a common way to reach audiences and potential consumer markets.[22] As a concept, the brand is tied to the person's sense of self, creating a relationship between the audience and the brand. *Concept brands* present niche audiences/markets with prepackaged symbols that enable consumers to express their lifestyles and dispositions in terms of a cultural system that is recognizable and easily communicated.[23] Just as the group of "career women in their thirties" can associate with the characters or story line of a television show and become part of that niche audience, Nike's concept brand can use similar associations to encourage women of this group to express themselves as active and diligent by wearing athletic shoes with the representative Nike swoosh.

In addition to individual attitudes, self-representation through the display of branded symbols and products can indicate group membership. Concept brands excel in this arena. The Benneton Corporation, a forerunner of this branding strategy, used non-traditional advertising campaigns from 1984 to 2000 that illustrated controversial social issues.[24] Benneton transformed issues from human rights to racism into imagery and symbolic expressions designed to elicit strong emotional responses from consumers. The ads never included Benneton's clothing at all, only the brand name. Affective brand recognition increased social awareness of the issue while constructing a new consumer identity rooted in symbolic commitment and conscientious consumption.[25] As a concept brand, Benneton produced a new niche audience with mass appeal, "the audience of the socially aware." Readers could view Benneton's ads, momentarily contemplate an important social issue, and think of ourselves as conscientious people. If we purchased Benneton's clothing, we could affirm our identity as members of this elite group every time we wore it. From social awareness derives conscientious consumption.

The color green to represent support for environmental conservation is a prime example of contemporary concept branding and conscientious consumption.[26] In response to international events, visible climate change, natural and man-made disasters, and increasingly limited natural resources, the growing concern for environmental issues, coupled with feelings of helplessness in the face of illness and death, has motivated many American consumers to think about what they can do to help. The answer: eco-friendly shopping. While the consumer-based approach to sustainability largely defines the mainstream environmental movement and appeals to millions of Americans, the niche market of the socially aware has enabled companies to foster a consumerist cultural identity oriented to social responsibility and individual lifestyle. In many social circles, it is fashionable to *Go Green*. Companies use stock imagery and green symbolism to promote green consumption and the public display of green lifestyle symbols. Neither the companies nor their products need to be environmentally friendly to use green symbolism to create the image of stylish social responsibility. Green itself functions as the concept brand. Any company or organization that uses it absorbs its meaning.

Similarly, it is fashionable to *Think Pink*. As King points out, strategic corporate philanthropy improves public relations and builds consumer loyalty while philanthropic consumption ignites consumers' desire to become more engaged citizens. These processes enable companies and organizations to create the impression that they are involved in public service first, and business second. They also facilitate the construction of a valued consumerist identity. Pink consumption draws upon the niche market/audience of the socially aware. Concept branding offers consumers an identity of social influence gained through a purchase, a lifestyle choice, or an affective brand association. In blurring the distinction between product and consumer, the branding process elevates the social importance of this valued cultural identity. The loyalties of the socially aware consumer go beyond specific corporate ties and instead support the concept, or in the case of breast cancer—*the cause*. Members of the breast cancer audience can see themselves as altruistic, conscientious, and socially aware whenever they buy or display pink.

WARRIORS IN PINK

The war metaphor in breast cancer representations provides a crucial framework for the breast cancer brand. Breast cancer is either a hidden enemy lurking in the darkness ready to attack when women least expect it, or it is a target on the battlefield for the she-ro (armed with optimism, culturally approved weaponry, and modern medicine) to strike down. The she-ro transforms in relation to the breast cancer audience she represents. As the Cancer Vixen, she is the diagnosed young woman who fights breast cancer with her feisty attitude and aggressive treatment. An ad for the cancer drug Arimidex depicts a woman wearing red boxing gloves, arms crossed against her chest.[27]

Infantilizing the she-ro to the status of a Power Puff Girl, a Precious Moments figure in pink shorts and a white tank top with the pink ribbon on it raises her little gloved fists above her head. The caption reads: "Life is worth fighting for."[28] But the she-ro need not be a diagnosed woman: feminine she-roism transfers to women at risk and supporters.

Ford Motor Company has capitalized on the she-ro's warrior imagery in its Warriors in Pink campaign. The 2007 campaign featured two-time Grammy-winner and former *American Idol* winner Kelly Clarkson as "the face" of the Warriors in Pink print campaign. Ford developed an official set of 14 "symbols of the warrior," which can be purchased from Ford's website as embroidered, iron-on patches for $8. Ford defines the meaning of each symbol: for instance, the Warriors symbol "represent[s] the powerful and courageous who fight against breast cancer;" the Angel Wings "honors the angels who have passed after their fight against breast cancer;" the Tree of Love "represents those who grow and stand tall together through adversity;" the Dove "represents the wish for quiet peace during the heat of battle;" the Crowned Warriors "remind us that breast cancer touches the lives of both genders." She-roes can display these warrior marks on their clothing, download them as wallpaper for their computers, purchase T-shirts, sweatshirts, caps, travel mugs, key rings, dog tags, car decals, vehicle magnets, and license frames with the warrior symbols.

The 2009 Ford Mustang with Warriors in Pink package was available on the Mustang coupe, convertible, and glass roof coupe.

The package includes a pink ribbon and pony fender badge, pink ribbon rocker tape and hood striping, charcoal leather trimmed seats with pink stitching, and charcoal floor mats with pink ribbon and contrast stitching. The limited-edition 2008 Mustang with Warriors in Pink package donated $250 per sale to Susan G. Komen for the Cure, totaling over $500,000. One of the 2008 Ford Mustangs was the pace car for a Komen race. The vehicle's owner said, "This car is a rolling billboard for the importance of breast cancer awareness…It is a phenomenal thing for Ford to do."[29] Yes, it is a billboard—for the breast cancer brand, for a specific version of awareness, for Ford Motor Company, and for the driver.

The Ford Mustang uses pink symbolism to evoke the breast cancer brand, and it works. "The pink ribbon is recognized everywhere she goes."[30] Ford's corporate partnership with the Komen Foundation equates "the cause" with Komen's mission, therefore circulating Komen's message that awareness means "early detection." According to Ford, the company has dedicated more than $90 million over the years in cash and in-kind donations. News stories and media deals publicize Ford's laudable corporate citizenship, something valuable to Ford during an industry slowdown, which has been "broader, deeper, and longer than previously expected."[31] Between 2005 and 2008, Ford reduced its salaried, hourly, and dealership personnel from 142,700 to 84,300.[32] Ford's commendable relationship with "the cause" offsets bad public relations stemming from the loss of salaries and healthcare for nearly 60,000 employees. It worked for the owner of the Komen pace car. Then again, maybe she doesn't know about Ford's motives, and for good reason.

Ford actively markets its relationship with the breast cancer cause, not its employee relations. In a section of Ford's Web site called "news articles," Ford does not actually provide news articles. Instead, it lists hyperlinks to public relations information, such as the "2007 Ford Warriors in Pink Campaign," which announces that "Ford reaches new audiences with their most comprehensive Warriors in Pink campaign yet in support of Susan G. Komen for the Cure."[33] Ford is aware of the power of the breast cancer audience: it provides an ever-expanding market for any company that advertises the breast cancer brand. The Ford Mustang is indeed a rolling billboard, one that accompanies a multipronged marketing campaign aimed at creating fervor around the war on breast cancer. The warriors in pink march forward to spread Komen's message, provide free advertisement for Ford, and represent themselves as conscientious, socially aware consumers.

As it operates in pink ribbon culture, the war metaphor provides a crucial platform for generating the primary associations at work in the breast cancer brand. These associations are the embodiment of the she-ro in the war against breast cancer. They concretize the dimensions of the breast cancer audience as survivors, women at risk, and supporters. And they provide a set of consistent messages for the mass dissemination of pink ribbon culture. These associations are visible in breast cancer advertisements, public service campaigns, community events, news articles, and breast cancer narratives. They draw on the social history of breast cancer, the broader cancer culture, pink femininity, and advocacy as well as contemporary marketing and branding processes. Breast cancer has been transformed from an important social issue to a lifestyle choice that is now available to anyone who displays the brand.

THE BREAST CANCER BRAND

The breast cancer brand, with the pink ribbon as its logo, draws from a uniform collection of images and meanings within pink ribbon culture. The brand uses a specific combination of information and experiences to create feelings and associations that forge a relationship between the concept and the niche audience/market. Breast cancer organizations, corporations, and individuals use the brand to increase "awareness," raise funds, and sell products and services. More importantly, the proliferation of the breast cancer brand increases the audience and transmits a cultural identity of social awareness to any person or entity associated with the brand. Pink ribbon culture and the breast cancer industry rely on the brand to disseminate a specific set of attitudes, traits, and beliefs that perpetuate breast cancer culture and promote the behaviors that fund them. Associating messages of fear, hope, and goodness with the concept of breast cancer stirs emotion and appeals to consumer motivation, ultimately perpetuating the brand and facilitating conscientious consumption as well as symbolic action.

Fear and the Pink Menace

Early depictions of breast cancer in women's magazines used fear of physical and/or social mutilation to promote breast examination and medical intervention as weapons in the war against breast cancer. In the 1940s and 1950s physicians and popular health magazines used imagery of women "blowing their brains out" to represent the seriousness of women's responsibility for breast examination to prevent cancer death.[34] A *Time* magazine article (1974) uses a similar image to promote women's personal responsibility for urgent medical intervention: "If a woman decides to go surgeon shopping and delays a couple of weeks, she's taking her life in her hands. You can't play Russian roulette with breast cancer." The new war on breast cancer is prettier, but no less urgent or aggressive. Popular magazines from 1980 to 1995 present breast cancer as frightening and seemingly unavoidable.[35] Fear of the inevitability and uncertainty of breast cancer impels urgent and aggressive action as quantified information about increasingly high incidence rates, high levels of recurrence, relatively flat mortality rates, and unavoidable risk factors (e.g., being a woman and getting older) suggest that all women should be afraid. Fear generates commitment to the war.

Urgency and aggressive action are synchronistic dimensions of fear in the breast cancer brand. RADO Switzerland is a high-end watch manufacturer advertising a pink watch fashioned in the shape of a breast cancer ribbon.[36] Next to the watch are the words "Time to Fight." The ad literally uses a timepiece to stress the urgency of the breast cancer war. In my analysis of 197 full-page breast cancer advertisements in four popular women's magazines from 1999 to 2007, 41 percent used "fighting" words to convey war, sporting competition, and the importance of aggressive action.[37] In an analysis of cancer reporting in the news, stories regularly highlight sports celebrities with cancer or everyday people with cancer who are involved in sports to convey a sense of heroic personal struggle.[38] Similarly, a tagline for Ford's Warrior Mustang emphasizes the importance of physical power in a competitive race: "Winning the race against breast cancer is going to take a whole lot of horsepower…The 2009 Ford Mustang with Warriors in Pink™ Package is adding more muscle to the fight."[39]

Sun Soy, an occasional sponsor of Komen Race events, uses sporting imagery to advertise its organic, non-dairy soy milk.[40] A 2002 advertisement during NBCAM portrays a fit woman in a racing jersey looking down with a pensive expression.[41] A large number on her racing bib reads: 203,500. Small text surrounds the number: "Because this year alone there will be 203,500 more reasons to fight breast cancer."

The bib number, resembling a racing number, signifies the number of new breast cancer cases predicted for the current year. The average reader may not know precisely that the American Cancer Society estimated 203,500 new cases of breast cancer in 2002, but it sounds right. The echo of such statistics across breast cancer representations grants authority to the statistic even as it reinforces fear and uncertainty about who these women will be. Contrasting the image of a young, healthy, and vibrant woman with frightening statistics emphasizes the association of fear, for even she is vulnerable to "this terrible disease."

For many women breast cancer *is* a terrible disease, and treatment for breast cancer often contributes to the horror of the experience. Many of the women I talked to in the past 8 years have described experiences I would not wish on anyone. The latter half of this book will share their voices. However, branding is not about the reality of women's experiences. The representations that circulate in cancer culture use simple associations to depict a narrow slice of reality that juxtaposes fear of breast cancer with hope and the goodness of the cause. The brand keeps the war going, but it does not represent the reality of breast cancer.

A frequent advertisement from Evelyn Lauder's Breast Cancer Research Foundation displays a fat pink eraser like those used in kindergarten. This eraser is etched with the breast cancer ribbon.[42] The words "Breast Cancer" at the center of the page are written in pencil and lightened as though they are beginning to be erased. Particles from the eraser sprinkle around the text and the parenthetic phrase "(erase it for good)" follows as a casual message that does not warrant the status of a full sentence. The informal tone is as welcoming as pink femininity. Bold, italicized lettering toward the bottom of the page reinforces the need for urgency and the presence of civilian casualties: "Breast cancer doesn't just affect women. Consider the families and friends whose lives are also changed." Statistics in smaller print lend legitimacy through quantification and call the reader to battle once again:

> In the US alone, 211,300 women and 1300 men will be diag-
> nosed with breast cancer this year, and 40,000 will die. We
> cannot rest until we win the battle against breast cancer. With
> your help, we can **erase this disease…for good"** [original
> emphasis]

The inevitability and uncertainty associated with breast cancer require urgent and aggressive action on the part of the entire breast cancer audience: the diagnosed, women at risk, and supporters (families and friends). Although this particular ad includes men in the statistics, the she-ro predominates in pink ribbon culture, not the hero.

Most representations of breast cancer use statistics to generate fear and the color pink to evoke innocence and femininity. In contrast to the pink ribbons that regularly pass through Esteé Lauder cosmetics counters, an advertisement for Evelyn Lauder's Breast Cancer Research Foundation uses a porous gray ribbon to denote the ominous and sinister nature of breast cancer.[43] The permeable aspect of the ribbon indicates vulnerability and ambiguity, while bold, large text reiterates the message that "Nobody is Safe. Yet." This attention-grabbing statement is a call for protection while it affirms the unknown future of breast cancer. Statistics once again reveal the prevalence of breast cancer while urging the reader to take action: "Join us in the fight against breast cancer." Such calls to arms saturate breast cancer representations, making the fear association an easily recognizable dimension of the breast cancer brand.

Hope and Faith in Breast Cancer Awareness

Hope provides a counter-balance to fear. Many advertisements use the word *hope*, and some pink ribbon products even use the word as a naming device, such as the limited-edition sculpture, the "Angel of Hope." Companies and organizations use an association with hope to generate feelings in potential audiences/consumers that will encourage them to participate in pink consumption and feel *hopeful* about what this might accomplish. Across representations, hope is often associated with optimism and a general sense of awareness. Just as in pink ribbon culture, optimism in ads takes the form of a positive outlook, courageous action, and the explicit omission of complaints. Awareness is tied to the visibility of breast cancer as a social problem through publicity and the proliferation of breast cancer symbols and products. Broad cultural scripts correspond to narratives and organizational processes in pink ribbon culture as consumers become transmitters of hope through voluntarism, social networking, pink consumption, and the giving of breast cancer products as gifts.

The pink ribbon represents breast cancer awareness, and the breast cancer brand uses awareness to generate hope. The general coupling of awareness and hope reinforces the brand and resonates with an audience who has been primed for the association with consistent and repeated messages in pink ribbon culture. An ad for the Komen Race for the Cure, for example, is written from the perspective of survivors. Beneath the image of a bald woman in a pink T-shirt, jewelry, and lipstick, the text reads: "We can live without our hair. We can live without our breasts. We cannot live without our hope for a cure."[44] The Avon Walk for Breast Cancer advertises hope as a counterpart to fear.[45] The words, "READY. SET. HOPE." take center stage. Similar to the refrain used to call the start of a race (ready, set, go), the sporting language suggests urgency and competition. Fortifying the message of hope is the line "For two days, we walk as one" and an array of photos featuring people who are hugging, holding hands, laughing, smiling, and wiping tears. Solidarity, emotion, and optimism lead to hope in the breast cancer race.

The largest photo in the Avon ad draws attention to two women looking directly at the camera. A generational age difference and subtle resemblance suggests a mother and daughter. In community walks breast cancer survivors, family members, and supporters often participate together. A head scarf beneath the older woman's pink survivor hat likely conceals hair loss resulting from chemotherapy. Her smile and participation signify hope for an active life after breast cancer treatment. Despite these hopeful images and words, there remains a sense of urgency. The small print mentions "the lives of millions affected by breast cancer," "under-insured women and men," and a "quest for a cure." Against this background, the words (Ready. Set.

Hope.) suggest that hope may be the best chance we have to win this race.

Breast cancer organizations disseminate hope with sentimentality and empowerment rhetoric used to encourage voluntarism and fundraising. Last year, the Komen Race for the Cure charged a $50 registration fee, and my local affiliate e-mailed frequent updates about the $500,000 fundraising goal (registration fee not included). An update of "important things to remember" described prize information, how to submit donations, and recruitment strategies.

- We encourage you to join in on the **Power of** 10 by asking 10 friends to donate $10 and then encourage your friends to then ask 10 of their friends to donate $10, and so on, and so on. (original emphasis)
- Don't forget to ask if your company has a matching program.

With hope in the background, this strategy emphasizes the participants' role in making choices and taking action. The organization defines the choices/action in terms of its agenda, and frames it in terms of em*power*ment. Participants voluntarily and enthusiastically take advantage of their personal networks to propagate the organization's messages, publicize the event, and raise funds. Although Komen's style of fundraising is common to a variety of causes, the breast cancer brand successfully blurs the line between advocacy and advertising through its use of culture.

Cultural representations of breast cancer are mutually rein-forcing, as media attention and cause-marketing strengthen the social force of the brand. Natrelle, maker of breast implants, capitalizes on the familiar hope association. A sparse and simple ad positions a nude woman on a white background, with her body in the shape of a ribbon.[46] The woman's upper body resembles the ribbon's loop, while her outstretched arms and legs cross to give the impression of its tails.

The caption reads: "Where there's awareness, there's hope." The lack of specificity begs the question: Awareness of what? The audi-ence already knows that the ribbon symbolizes breast cancer aware-ness, and hope has already been linked to awareness across the brand and throughout pink ribbon culture. After stating in the fine print that the company supports Susan G. Komen for the Cure, Natrelle urges the reader to "learn more about breast reconstruction options with the *Natrelle* Collection." The association of hope vis-à-vis awareness is tied to Komen's name recognition, fusing hope with visibility. The nude female form is a literal embodiment of this message. She also presents a woman whose femininity, sexuality, and desirability *are* intact.[47] Not only is there hope that she will survive breast cancer, there is hope that with awareness of Natrelle's prod-ucts she can return to her original feminine state after treatment.

Goodness, Fundraising, and the Pink Lifestyle

The breast cancer brand consistently conveys its associations across awareness promotions, fundraising campaigns, products, and services. During NBCAM (and throughout the year) pink ribbons and products abound in supermarkets, shopping malls, magazines, newspapers, television shows, billboards, and workplaces with inspirational stories from pink ribbon culture to accompany them. The association of pink goodness creates an association with innocence, femininity, and virtue while disassociating with marginal lifestyle choices. The media-friendly interplay of pink femininity and the broader cancer culture provides a light, entertaining, and at times comical depiction. A streaming video on NBCAM's Web site uses clay animation of a talking pink ribbon with large lips and eyelashes. The ribbon, with a child-like voice, flies from one office cubicle to the next, first to tell a African American woman, and then a white woman, that "early detection saves lives…get a mammogram every year…Tell your friends!" Emphasizing brand dissemination through social networks, the animated ribbon makes breast cancer palatable while enforcing the role of mammography screening in solving the breast cancer problem. The "pink kitsch" produces visibility and offsets fear.

The brand encourages individuals and corporations to support the cause through consumption and social networking. Mass media offers representation for those who participate. Active members of the breast cancer audience are cast as good, great, generous, committed, and doing their part. Ads for an Avon Breast Cancer Walk characterize the people and the event: "GREAT PEOPLE" and "GREAT WEEKEND."[48] The women's head scarves indicate that they are survivors. They are smiling triumphantly—the message is, if these women can walk, then so can you. Similar to other "thons," the breast cancer walks correlate moral worth, volunteerism, and individual responsibility for one's health (i.e., "Doing good by running well"[49]). Those who take part (individuals and corporations) build a civic identity based in consumption and symbolic commitment.

In addition to supporting a good cause, pink consumption can be an enjoyable and satisfying lifestyle choice. Avon asks readers directly, "When was the last time you had a really GREAT WEEKEND?" (original emphasis). The focus is on personal fulfillment that aligns with a pink lifestyle. Another Avon ad reads: "Good things come to those who WALK."[50] In other words, good people who do something good will receive good things in return. This sentiment once again calls upon the reader to reflect on his or her values and actions. Consistently, images of happy people engaging in fun activities suggest that good things come to those who *pink*.

The pink lifestyle necessitates pink consumption. A four-page ad in *Self* magazine for the "Cure Card" reads: "Tell your mom, sister, and best friend—it's time to go shopping…Get special offers, discounts, and more from your favorite retailers and brands…Discounts Galore…So go ahead…Treat Yourself to the Cure Card."[51] The Cure Card associates breast cancer with the innocence of a mother, sister, and best friend even as it identifies retailers as good corporate citizens who provide consumers with the opportunities to do something good. The Cure Card depicts pink consumption and lifestyle as enjoyable, easy, and rewarding. The word *treat* suggests indulgence, while alluding to the treat*ment* that proceeds may help to provide. When the going gets tough, the women go shopping! Such ads target the women shoppers who make up the magazine's audience, thereby extending the reach of pink ribbon culture and reinforcing women's normative roles as consumers.[52] The breast cancer brand encourages consumers to treat themselves to the vast selection of pink products and feel-good activities in support of the cause.

To keep hope (and the brand) alive, corporations tie their marketing strategies to breast cancer advocacy, which provides justification for corporate and consumer interest. Ford's Tied to the Cause campaign covered the pages of women's magazines from 2000 to 2006: "The campaign features a commemorative bandanna...to promote Ford's breast cancer awareness campaign and longstanding relationship with the Susan G. Komen Breast Cancer Foundation's Race for the Cure[(R)] Series."[53] The prominent breast cancer organization supplies legitimacy and reminds the reader of the seriousness of breast cancer. In addition, Ford does not have to modify its own brand associations because pink symbolism evokes the breast cancer brand's readily available and easily recognizable associations. (The campaign displays the familiar Ford emblem next to or centered atop a pink ribbon.) The campaign uses star power to highlight the pink lifestyle, featuring celebrities (such as Demi Moore, Cuba Gooding Jr., Yasmine Bleeth, Sarah Michele Geller, Mary J. Blige, the stars from the television show *ER*, and others) wearing the limited-edition silk scarf (retail price, $35).[54] The individuals, their sponsors, and Ford glean recognition, social acceptance, and good will through their affiliation with the good cause of breast cancer. Even without mention of awareness or research, pink symbolism and lifestyle are sufficient to convey the breast cancer brand and provide the proper associations.

Pink lifestyle enables consumers to do good for a good cause, with status and style. A fashionable person can shop for the cure, laugh for the cure, drink wine for the cure, buy shoes for the cure, listen to music for the cure, get a massage for the cure, spend a weekend in a fancy hotel for the cure, test-drive a BMW for the cure, or use their *pink tech* for the cure. An ad for the Laugh Out Loud Comedy Benefit for Breast Cancer Awareness features four notable women comedians and bright colors and uses the hip Internet slang LOL! to describe the fun and trendy outing.[55] Brand associations stir emotions that encourage some to take action—even if the action is symbolic (e.g., "Tune in, and just imagine what you'll save!"[56]). Symbolic action is the ultimate consequence of concept branding: imagination replaces action. Media representations foster a representational relationship between the media consumer and the breast cancer brand. Warriors in pink can *think pink* or occasionally *do pink*, while they are represented in mass media and pink ribbon culture as good people who support a good cause. As a member of the niche market of the socially aware, any consumption—of products, services, or mass-mediated ideas—is enough to construct an identity as a conscientious consumer. Once incorporated into cultural identity, loyalty to the brand surpasses any particular consumer transaction.

The mediated cultural environment within which pink ribbon culture operates facilitates the branding of breast cancer. The branding process positions the cause to become more than a health topic or social problem. Breast cancer is now a vital lifestyle choice available to anyone who displays the brand. The proliferation of the brand through mass media enables individuals to form a representational bond with breast cancer as a concept. Consumers' emotional responses to the brand associations encourage a cultural identity based on seeing oneself as a member of the niche market of the socially aware. This cultural identity constructs a loyal relationship with the brand that bolsters social support for breast cancer as a good and important cause. With this support comes greater opportunity for the consumption of breast cancer products, services, and lifestyles. Media consumers engage in real or symbolic action on behalf of breast cancer through the associative feelings and beliefs that the brand evokes. After two decades of cause-marketing, the breast cancer brand exists in its own right, with little (or less) regard to the sponsoring entity.

KOMEN'S NEW LOGO

The pink ribbon is a generic symbol in the public domain, which cannot be owned or controlled by a single entity; any individual, organization, or corporation can use the pink ribbon as a visual

cue to signify breast cancer awareness. Breast cancer organizations argue that the pink ribbon is a visual symbol that prompts
people to discuss breast cancer, educate themselves, and take
action. This may be so. However, the breast cancer brand has
also facilitated a shift in the functioning of the pink ribbon
from a disease-specific symbol to a brand logo. Organizations
and corporations, regardless of tax status, donate to breast
cancer organizations or programs through product sales or
fundraising events. In addition to promoting good will, public
relations, and charitable tax deductions, the branding of breast
cancer maintains the status of breast cancer as a social problem,
encourages pink consumption, and sustains the brand, its audience, and its primary associations. The branding process produces attitudes, dispositions, and beliefs that uphold pink
ribbon culture and consolidate its power in American society.

To distinguish itself from other breast cancer organizations,
the Susan G. Komen Breast Cancer Foundation changed its
name to Susan G. Komen for the Cure in 2007. According to
Komen, "The name change was accompanied by a new brand
image. The new logo included a pink `running ribbon' designed
specifically for Komen for the Cure." Komen used an advertising
campaign to introduce the new ribbon as a registered trademark
and set it apart from generic pink ribbons. In one ad the Running
Ribbon is fashioned into the letter "I" as the reader is asked to
"[I]magine life without breast cancer." The ad reads:

> *Imagine* the day when survivors like Becky Gabriele won't have to
> *fear* for the lives of their daughters...That's the *vision* we all share.

And with *your help*, this is the *ribbon* that will make it a reality. Visit ThisIsThe Ribbon.org." (emphasis added)

Even with a new logo, the breast cancer brand remains intact through its associations: fear (for the lives of their daughters), hope (through imagination and Komen's vision), and goodness (achieved with your help and the new Komen ribbon). Yet Komen declares that its new ribbon is different. A press release states that the new ribbon:[57]

> signifies the promise Komen Founder Nancy G. Brinker made to her dying sister, Susan G. Komen, to do what she could to end breast cancer. Today, any generic pink ribbon can be used to represent breast cancer awareness while the Komen 'running ribbon' is reserved solely for use by Susan G. Komen for the Cure®.

Komen clearly understands the importance of image in contemporary culture. The stylized pink ribbon looks different from other ribbons, but it supports the same breast cancer brand. So, why did Komen trademark a new logo?

The breast cancer brand operates in a culture that is commerce-based and mass-mediated, designed to sell products, services, and a way of life to an ever-expanding audience base. Thus, the brand relies on self-referential reinforcement from pink ribbon culture and the broader media system. As distinctions between print, broadcast, entertainment, and Web-based media continue to blur, brand associations are necessarily simple and superficial. In most cases, those who circulate the brand are not held accountable for the accuracy, relevance, or completeness of the informational sound bites they disseminate, or their outcomes. Their associations and symbolism foster brand recognition and consumer loyalty, while shaping public commitment. The organizations at the center of pink ribbon culture define the means for addressing breast cancer as a social problem.

As the most widely known and best-funded breast cancer organization in the United States, Komen has the greatest number of corporate partnerships (over 200) and leads in revenue from corporate cause-marketing campaigns. Komen's assets increased from $109.3 million in 2003 to $316.9 million in 2007.[58] Brand image helps the organization to maintain its leading position in pink ribbon culture. The organization uses contemporary marketing strategies common in commerce and mass media to target its audience through word of mouth, advertising, interactions with organizational representatives, and real-life experiences. Advertising is a growing component of this strategy. Komen's financial statements report $52.6 million in contributed goods and services for the year ending March 31, 2007, primarily related to local television, radio, and newspaper advertising for the Race Series events. Because of the special role of women's magazines in the history of breast cancer, Komen also advertises widely in women's magazines. The foundation incurred advertising expenses of approximately $41.8 million in 2007, the majority of which was contributed.[59] In addition, the organization gets free advertising every time an entity uses Komen's name to affiliate with the breast cancer cause. With brand associations intact, Komen's quest to define the trademarked Running Ribbon as the authentic logo for the breast cancer brand enables Komen to dominate the breast cancer market and pink ribbon culture. This is *the* ribbon.

NOTES

1. L. Belkin, "How Breast Cancer Became This Year's Hot Charity," *The New York Times Magazine*, December 22, 1996: 46.

2. S. King, *Pink Ribbons, Inc.: Breast Cancer and the Politics of Philanthropy* (Minneapolis: University of Minnesota Press, 2006), vii.

3. M. E. Zuckerman, *A History of Popular Women's Magazines in the United States, 1792–1995* (Westport, CT: Greenwood Press, 1998).

4. M. W. Flexner, "Cancer—I've Had It," *Ladies' Home Journal* 57 (May 1947): 150, quoted in B. Lerner, *The Cancer Wars: Hope, Fear, and the Pursuit of a Cure in Twentieth-Century America* (New York: Oxford University Press, 2001), 44.

5. G. Palmer, "I Had Cancer," *Ladies' Home Journal* 64 (July 1947): 143-8, 150, 152-3, quoted in Lerner, *The Cancer Wars*.

6. "Self-Examination of the Breasts," *Good Housekeeping* (November 1955): 32, quoted in Lerner, *The Cancer Wars.*

7. D. Emerson, "Cancer and a Woman's Sex," *Woman's Home Companion* January (1955), 28.

8. B. Ehrenreich & D. English, *For Her Own Good: 150 Years of the Expert's Advice to Women* (New York: Anchor Books, 1978).

9. E. Leopold, *A Darker Ribbon: Breast Cancer, Women, and Their Doctors in the Twentieth Century* (Boston, MA: Beacon Press, 1999): 122-3.

10. J. Ramsey, "A Healthier Bosom," *Ladies' Home Journal* April (1969), 82, quoted in J. A. Karran Fosket & C. LaFia, "Breast Cancer in Popular Women's Magazines from 1913 to 1996," in *Breast Cancer: Society Shapes an Epidemic*, eds. A. Kaspar & S. Ferson, 303-24 (New York: St. Martin's Press, 2000). Magazines in the sample include *Good Housekeeping, Ladies' Home Journal, Woman's Home Companion, Cosmopolitan, Vogue, Redbook, Ms., Mademoiselle, Glamour, Harper's Bazaar,* and *Working Woman.*

11. B. Jones, "Courage That Runs in the Family," *Good Housekeeping,* May 19, 1996, quoted in J. Clarke, "A Comparison of Breast, Testicular and Prostate Cancer in Mass Print Media (1996–2001)," *Social Science and Medicine* 59, no. 3 (2003): 541-51.

12. S. T. Black, "Don't Sit Home and Be Afraid," *McCall's* February (1973): 82-83, 114-6; G. Caplan, "An Outpouring of Love for Shirley Temple Black," *McCall's* March (1973): 48-54, in Lerner, *The Cancer Wars.*

13. B. Ford, "Breast Cancer Fear and Facts," *Time,* November 4, 1974.

14. J. L. Andsager & A. Powers, "Social or Economic Concerns: How News and Women's Magazines Framed Breast Cancer in the 1990s," *Journal and Mass Communication Quarterly* 76, no. 3 (1999): 531-50.

15. V. Freimuth, R. Greenberg, J. DeWitt, R. M. Romano, et al., "Covering Cancer: Newspapers and the Public Interest," *Journal of Communication,* 34 (1984), 62-73.

16. The number of women with breast cancer nearly doubled between 1970 and 1990.

17. From 1987 to 1990 alone, there was a 33 percent increase in articles on breast cancer. See K. K. Gerlach, C. Marino, D. L. Weed, et al., "Lack of Colon Cancer Coverage in Seven Women's Magazines," *Women & Health* 26 (Summer 1997): 57-68.

18. E. Leopold, *A Darker Ribbon*, 123.

19. D. Croteau & W. Hoynes, *Media/Society: Industries, Images, and Audiences* (Thousand Oaks, CA: Pine Forge Press, 2003).

20. American Cancer Society, *Cancer Facts and Figures* 2008 (Atlanta: American Cancer Society, 2008).

21. "About Us," National Breast Cancer Awareness Month. http://nbcam.org/about_nbcam.cfm; K. Miller, "AstraZeneca and Breast Cancer Advocacy," *Breast Disease* 10, nos. 5 and 6 (1998): 67-70.

22. A. Jannson, "The Mediatization of Consumption: Towards an Analytical Framework of Image Culture," *Journal of Consumer Culture* 21 (2002): 5-31; E. Moor, "Branded Spaces: The Scope of 'New Marketing,'" *Journal of Consumer Culture* 31 (2003): 39-60; S. Nandan, "An Exploration of the Brand Identity-Brand Image Linkage: A Communications Perspective," *Journal of Brand Management* 124 (2005): 264-78; C. W. Park, B. J. Jaworski, & D. J. MacInnis, "Strategic Brand Concept-Image Management," *Journal of Marketing* 50 (1986): 135-45.

23. J. A. Howard & J. N. Sheth, *The Theory of Buyer Behavior* (New York: John Wiley & Sons, 1969); A. Jannson, "The Mediatization of Consumption"; J. Connolly & A. Prothero, "Green Consumption: Life-Politics, Risk and Contradictions," *Journal of Consumer Culture* 91 (2008): 117-45; E. Rochberg-Halton, "Object Relations, Role Models, and Cultivation of the Self," *Environment and Behavior* 163 (1984): 335-68.

24. H. Giroux, "Consuming Social Change: The 'United Colors of Benetton,'" *Cultural Critique* (Winter 1994): 5-32.

25. G. H. Bower & J. P. Forgas, "Mood and Social Memory," in *The Handbook of Affect and Social Cognition*, ed. J. P. Forgas, 95-120 (Mahway, NJ: Erlbaum, 2001).

26. Connolly and Prothero, "Green Consumption."

27. Arimidex advertisement, *Ladies' Home Journal* October (2003): 180-1.

28. Precious Moments advertisement, *Self* October (2000): 193.

29. T. Dahduli, "Warriors in Pink: Driving for the Cure," *The Lasso* (October 23, 2008): 1.

30. *Ibid.*

31. "Company Reports: Financial Results 2008 Q3 Financial Results," Ford Motor Company, http://www.ford.com/about-ford/investor-relations/company-reports.

32. *Ibid.*

33. "2007 Ford Warriors in Pink Campaign," Ford Motor Company. http://www.fordvehicles.com/warriorsinpink/wip/article/?aid=9.

34. F. S. Slaughter, *The New Science of Surgery* (New York: Julian Messner, 1946), 244, quoted in Lerner, *The Cancer Wars.*

35. P. Lantz & K. Booth, "The Social Construction of the Breast Cancer Epidemic," *Social Science and Medicine* 46, no. 7 (1998): 907-18.

36. RADO Switzerland, "Time to Fight," *Self* October (2007): 145.

37. G. Sulik & A. Deane, "Coping in Pink: Representations of Breast Cancer Support and Survivorship in Women's Magazines," (paper presented at the American Sociological Association Annual Meeting, Sheraton Boston and the Boston Marriott Copley Place, Boston, MA, July 31, 2008).

38. C. Seale, "Sporting Cancer: Struggle Language in News Reports of People with Cancer," *Sociology of Health and Illness* 233 (2001): 308-29.

39. "Warrior Mustang," Ford Motor Company, http://www.fordvehicles.com/warriorsinpink/mustang/.

40. "Sun Soy sponsors breast cancer fundraiser," Nutraingredients.com, http://www.nutraingredients.com/Consumer-Trends/Sun-Soy-sponsors-breast-cancer-fundraiser.

41. "Sun Soy," *Self* October (2002): 147.

42. "The Breast Cancer Research Foundation," *Essence* October (2003): 133.

43. Breast Cancer Research Foundation, "Nobody is Safe. Yet." *Self* October (1994): 100.

44. "Komen Race for the Cure," *Fitness* November (2004): 75.

45. "Avon Walk for Breast Cancer," *Self* October (2007): 163.

46. "Natrelle," *Self* October (2007): 195.

47. M. Klawiter, "Breast Cancer in Two Regimes: The Impact of Social Movements on Illness Experience," *Sociology of Health & Illness* 26 (September 2004): 845-74.

48. "Avon Walk for Breast Cancer," *Self* October (2004): 121; "Avon Walk for Breast Cancer," *Self* January (2004): 79; "Avon Walk for Breast Cancer," *Self* November (2004): 133.

49. S. King, *Pink Ribbons, Inc.: Breast Cancer and the Politics of Philanthropy* (Minneapolis: University of Minnesota Press, 2006), 29.

50. "Avon Breast Cancer Walk, "Good Things Come to Those Who Walk," *Self* January (2006): 79.

51. "The Cure Card," *Self* December (2004): 105-8.

52. K. Breazeale, "In Spite of Women: *Esquire* Magazine and the Construction of the Male Consumer," *Signs* (1994): 1-22; C. Frederick, *Selling Mrs. Consumer* (New York: Business Bourse, 1929).

53. PR Newswire, "Ford and Lilly Pulitzer 'Tie Up' to Fight Breast Cancer," news release, May 8, 2003.

54. Ford Motor Company, "A Real-Life Emergency," *Essence* October (2005): 114-5.

55. "Laugh Out Loud Comedy Show," *Self* October (2007): 135.

56. "Tune In and Just Imagine What You'll Save."

57. Susan G. Komen for the Cure, "The Pink Ribbon Story," http://ww5.komen.org/uploadedFiles/Content_Binaries/The_Pink_Ribbon_Story.pdf.

58. The Susan G. Komen Breast Cancer Foundation, Inc. dba Susan G. Komen for the Cure and Affiliates, "Consilidated Financial Statements

Years Ended March 31, 2004 and 2003," http://ww5.komen.org/uploaded Files/Content_Binaries/2003-2004finalauditedfinancial.pdf; The Susan G. Komen Breast Cancer Foundation, Inc. dba Susan G. Komen for the Cure and Affiliates, "Consilidated Financial Statements Years Ended March 31, 2007 and 2006," http://ww5.komen.org/AboutUs/Financial Information.html.

59. Susan G. Komen Breast Cancer Foundation, "Consolidated Financial Statements Years Ended March 31, 2007 and 2006."

FIVE

CONSUMING MEDICINE,
SELLING SURVIVORSHIP

*By virtue of growing up in a culture where cancer is characterized
as the ultimate enemy invading the body; where the body becomes
battleground, split from the mind that must become a disembodied
warrior; where the patient becomes a soldier, entreated to
follow absolutely the orders of the heroic medical professional;
and where an aggressive, search and destroy strategy often
inflicts more damage than the foe, the [patients'] experience is
virtually predetermined.*

KRISTEN GARRISON, "THE PERSONAL IS RHETORICAL"[1]

O ver the historical course of the breast cancer movement,
activists emphasized breast cancer as a women's health
epidemic to stir public interest and deepen social investment in
the cause. This investment grew in the midst of an existing
cancer culture that favored the war metaphor. Images of swords
and shields, fighting words and slogans, and volunteer collectivi-
ties led to an eventual *declaration of war* on cancer in 1971 when
Richard Nixon enacted the National Cancer Act (NCA).[2] The
purpose of the NCA was to enlarge the authorities of the
National Cancer Institute (NCI) and the National Institutes
of Health (NIH) to advance the general effort against cancer.

This effort was defined as an "effective attack" through the use of "all of the biomedical resources of the National Institutes of Health" (NCA, Section 2). The war on cancer undeniably influenced the biomedical treatment of breast cancer, as the desire to fight and win included radical surgery, toxic radiation and chemotherapy, and controversies within the medical system itself about what constituted evidence of effective treatment.

The logic that resulted from the war declaration was that if women were to feel empowered to take action in the war against breast cancer, they needed a well-funded infrastructure that included weapons, strategies, commanding officers, and heroic role models. Inadvertently or not, the developing pink ribbon culture provided that infrastructure. Uniting modern medicine and the cancer industry within a cultural system that would promote medical consumerism in tandem with hopeful communities of survivorship, pink ribbon culture created a new archetype for diagnosed women. Maren Klawiter describes the modern breast cancer survivor as "a woman who had struggled bravely and victoriously against the disease (which, ideally, was diagnosed early, due to her disciplined practice of "breast health" and rigorous observation of screening guidelines), and whose survival was therefore assured."[3] Cultivating the belief in early detection, faith in the medical system, and a fervent commitment to medical consumerism, the triumphant survivor (she-ro) would promote medical surveillance and intervention with renewed hope for a future without breast cancer. As the war rages on, pink ribbon culture strives to keep hope alive.

Breast cancer rates have increased about 1 percent per year since the 1940s. However, since 1982 the breast cancer incidence in women aged 40 years and above has been increasing at a much faster rate.[4] According to the NCI, breast cancer rates increased by more than 40 percent from 1973 to 1998. The NCI estimated 250,230 new cases of breast cancer in 2008, up from 192,200 in 2001. About 77 percent of these cases are "invasive" (have the capacity to spread), and for at least a third of diagnosed women the disease eventually does spread. While 75 percent of recurrences happen within 5 years, 25 percent occur after the 5-year period. About 35 percent of breast cancer patients who have metastatic disease at diagnosis (stage 3 or 4, when the cancer has already spread beyond the primary site) tend to live 5 years or longer.[5] Breast cancer remains the second leading cause of cancer death for women, after lung cancer, and is the leading cause of cancer death for women between the ages of 20 and 59, and for Hispanic women as a whole at any age. Each year over 40,000 American women die from the disease.[6] Although the United States spends billions of dollars a year to fight breast cancer, there are still no proven methods of prevention, and there is no cure. The absolute risk of dying from breast cancer has decreased about 0.05 percent from 1990 to 2005. Yet a woman diagnosed with invasive breast cancer gets more treatment, spends more money, and has the about the same chances of dying from the disease as she did 50 years ago. Why aren't we winning the war?

THE BREAST CANCER INDUSTRY

The force of profitability of breast cancer detection and treatment cannot be ignored as a key element of society's failure to eradicate breast cancer. In a capitalistic society, financial incentives facilitate progress. Without financial incentives, progress is slow and sometimes utterly impossible. This is not news. The war on breast cancer thrives within a consumer-minded, ever-expanding healthcare industry that is one of the largest and fastest-growing sectors of the U.S. economy. Healthcare has risen from 7.2 percent of the gross domestic product (GDP) in 1965 to over 16 percent of GDP today, and it is projected to increase to 20 percent of GDP by 2015 to total over $4 trillion in health expenditures.[7] Per-person health spending has also been increasing at faster rates in recent years, from $144 per capita in 1960 to almost $4,400 in 1999, and to $7,110 in 2006. By 2015, the cost per person for health expenses is projected to increase to $12,320.[8] While the question of how to reduce healthcare costs and provide access to quality care is a concern for medical practitioners, consumers, and advocates alike as well as a subject of heated national debate, profit centers within the cancer industry continue to expand medical markets and encourage medical consumption.[9]

Understanding economic incentives requires analyzing how economic forces work to build and maintain institutions—in this case, the cancer industry. The economic incentives of the cancer industry help to create a consumer-oriented environment that shapes the medical and scientific enterprise. Paul Starr's classic history of medicine, for example, traces the origins in the 1900s of our current allopathic medical system to an alliance with drug producers, who remain the source of drug information for our physicians.[10] Professional socialization within this environment contributes to the beliefs, protocols, and practices that keep the industry going. For example, the treatment and eradication of breast cancer is a stated goal for many in the medical and scientific professions. Despite these good intentions, most individuals necessarily operate within the cancer industry, which places a high value on market share and profit. Customers guarantee sales, revenue, research streams, employment, and industry growth. The social and clinical investment in diseases with large markets (e.g., women at risk for, or diagnosed with, breast cancer) supplies a huge number of customers for a broad range of cancer-related products and services.

In 1996, breast cancer incidence had already risen substantially in the United States and the breast cancer movement had begun to succeed in rallying political support and public interest. At this juncture, medical doctor John Lee and biochemist David Zava published *What Your Doctor May Not Tell You About Breast Cancer*, which sold close to 875,000 copies. The book, which extended earlier treatises on the cancer industry such as Samuel Epstein's (1979) *The Politics of Cancer*[11] and Ralph W. Moss's (1980) *The Cancer Syndrome*,[12] argued that the history and politics of the market-based breast cancer industry were the fundamental reasons we were unable to identify the causes of breast cancer, prevent the disease, or find an ultimate cure. Its candid statements were startling to many. Since there was no improvement in mortality rates from breast cancer from 1930 on, the examples just made sense: "All those mammograms, biopsies, lumpectomies, and mastectomies, and all that chemotherapy, radiation, and tamoxifen create a substantial income stream for hospitals, physicians, their support staff, those who make all the equipment, and especially those who make the drugs. And that doesn't even take into consideration all the research being done that's funded by [what is now billions of]...dollars donated to nonprofit breast cancer organizations."

By implicating the breast cancer industry and its politics in the failure of the medical system to do anything meaningful to eradicate breast cancer, the book drew attention to the limits of conventional medicine, accusing it of becoming strangled by market-based logic. The 2002 edition stated, once again, that "conventional medicine has done very little to make any meaningful difference in what will happen to you if you get breast cancer, and virtually nothing it has done has reduced the incidence of the disease."[13] Lee and Zava were hoping for a revolution. The revised edition came out at a critical time in the social history of breast cancer, when American women were alarmed to learn that their trust in the system may have been misplaced: the results of the 2002 Women's Health Initiative had just shown that the widely prescribed hormone replacement therapy drugs (HRT) were responsible for a significant portion of breast cancer cases, without the assumed heart benefits promoted by drug companies and well-meaning physicians. With the strength of the women's health and breast cancer movements, along with publicity about HRT as an industry failure, the time was right for American women to fight the cancer industry if they wanted to fight breast cancer.

There were small and repeated uprisings, but there was no revolution—at least not in pink ribbon culture. The details and politics of the breast cancer industry continued to be carefully hidden beneath war rhetoric, official policy, medical protocol and authority, pink ribbon culture, corporate interests, and a market-driven healthcare system. Devra Davis's, *The Secret History of the War on Cancer,* shows how public health campaigns have consistently overlooked and even suppressed data about cancer's systemic causes to keep profits flowing for a variety of private sectors.[14] The flurry of activity that surrounds the cause of breast cancer today still camouflages how the breast cancer industry profits from the war—from disease classification, medical technology and equipment, drug manufacturing and delivery, and industry ties to advocacy. These factors fuel the breast cancer industry, contributing both to its financial growth and to the losing war on breast cancer.

DISEASE CLASSIFICATION

Cancer, broadly defined, is a disease of abnormal cell growth, which occurs in some organs or tissues of the body at different rates, and either may be contained in a single mass (tumor) or may spread to other locations in the body (malignancy). It is the combination of abnormal cell growth and the ability to spread that makes cancer dangerous.[15] Yet some cancers are more dangerous than others. The assessment of just how dangerous a particular cancer may be is based on a disease classification system that begins with the tissue and cell type from which the cancer arises. Beyond this, there is little public understanding about what accounts for significant differences in the level of threat that a particular type of cancer may pose to the person diagnosed. Without much distinction, the "C" word in American culture signifies an embodied war that, if fought aggressively and valiantly with the tools of modern medicine and the power of positive thinking, can be won—casualties notwithstanding.

Beyond the basic definition and generalized belief about what cancer is lies a more detailed and complex classification system, which has stirred considerable controversy in the medical community. The first order of classification is based on cell type. Breast cancer is made up of abnormal breast cells. However, there are critical differences in classification based on whether these abnormal cells appear in the ducts (tubes that carry milk to the nipple) or the lobules (glands that make milk) and, more importantly, whether these abnormal cells have the capacity to spread (metastasize). Metastasis is what makes cancer life-threatening. The specific constellation of these features helps to categorize nine different breast conditions, some of which are called cancer. The following discussion will give the reader an understanding of why there is controversy about which of these breast conditions should be classified as a breast cancer, and the importance of disease classification for the growth and maintenance of the breast cancer industry.

(For a comprehensive discussion of breast cancer classifications and related terms, readers should seek out *Dr. Susan Love's Breast Book*, which *The New York Times* and many diagnosed women refer to as "The bible for women with breast cancer.")

The most important distinguishing characteristic among breast cancer types is whether they are *in situ*, or invasive. *In situ*, meaning "in place," is a term that specifies a tumor that is confined to the immediate area where it began. If a cluster of abnormal cells remains confined to the ducts, it is called ductal carcinoma *in situ* (DCIS). If the abnormal cells are confined to the lobules, it is called lobular carcinoma *in situ* (LCIS). Both conditions are asymptomatic and nearly always nonpalpable (cannot be felt by hand), and the abnormal cells do not invade surrounding breast tissue or spread to other parts of the body. *Invasive* (sometimes called *infiltrating*) is a term that signifies abnormal cells originating either in the lining of the ducts and invading nearby breast tissue (invasive ductal carcinoma), or that start in the lobules and break into nearby breast tissue (invasive lobular carcinoma). Invasive types, which represent the majority of breast cancers in the United States (77 percent), are the most dangerous because they have the capacity to invade blood and lymph vessels and spread to other parts of the body. Of the 250,230 new cases of breast cancer among women in 2008, the NCI estimated that there were 182,460 cases of invasive breast cancers and (detectable now with mammograms) 67,770 *in situ* cases. There is a wide range of disagreement about how to classify, and thereby treat, these less frequent *in situ* types.

DCIS, representing 85 percent of *in situ* diagnoses, is at the center of an ongoing debate. The term *carcinoma* refers to cancer (i.e., malignant tumor). Carcinoma is a misnomer for an *in situ* cluster of abnormal cells that seems to lack the capacity to metastasize.[16] In fact, in a 2008 editorial in the *Journal of the National Cancer Institute*, Drs. H. Gilbert Welch, Steven Woloshin, and Lisa M. Schwartz acknowledged that "a senior pathologist involved in developing classification systems confided to one of [them] that he regretted the use of the term carcinoma in DCIS."[17] More accurately, DCIS is a breast condition that can be a *precursor* to invasive breast cancer, or it can be a *risk factor* for the development of an invasive breast cancer at some point in the future. Differing views among doctors about whether to refer to DCIS as a cancer in clinical practice reflect the mismatch between name and definition. An oncologist at the Dana-Farber Cancer Institute and Brigham and Women's Hospital in Boston, Dr. Ann Partridge, reported at the 2005 San Antonio Breast Cancer Symposium that while 40 percent of doctors "always" refer to DCIS as cancer, 22 percent of doctors "never" or "almost never" do.[18]

The DCIS naming problem reflects a deeper issue, which Welch and colleagues point out in their *JNCI* editorial. DCIS represents a "big gray zone" between normal tissue and invasive cancer. No one knows which clusters of abnormal cells will progress to cancer and which ones will not, or which women diagnosed with the condition will develop an invasive cancer elsewhere in their breasts sometime in the future and which ones will not. The 2005 report from Partridge and colleagues also illustrated this lack of clarity, revealing differences in doctors' perceptions of risk related to DCIS. While 63 percent of doctors rated DCIS as a "1" or "2" on a 5-point risk scale, 36 percent rated the risk as a "3" or "4."[19] The naming problem, coupled with the inability to accurately assess the probable outcomes of DCIS, either as a pre-cancer or as a risk factor, leads to two crucial questions. First, is DCIS as dangerous as a cancer? Second, should DCIS be treated as if it were a cancer?

Cancer's threat is determined through staging, which is based on the size of the original tumor, level of lymph node involvement, and whether the cancer has metastasized (spread) to other parts of the body. On average, 61 percent of breast cancers are diagnosed at stage 1 (when they are localized to the primary site); 31 percent are diagnosed at stage 2 or 3 (when the cancer has spread beyond the primary site or to regional lymph nodes, but not to other organs); and 6 percent are diagnosed at stage 4 (when the cancer, as detected by lymph node dissection and computed tomography [CT] scans, is metastatic and has spread beyond the primary site to regional lymph nodes or to other organs of the body such as the lungs, liver, bones, or brain).[20] At stage 4, treatment tends to be more aggressive, and the survival rate at 5 years is about 20 percent, compared to 76 to 88 percent for stage 2.[21]

The difference in average survival rates at 5 years drives the push to detect breast cancer at earlier stages. However, staging cannot be understood separately from disease classification. DCIS is classified as a stage 0 cancer because it is contained to the primary site, cannot spread, and does not tend to become cancer. Level of threat: low. Because doctors are unable to determine which individuals who have DCIS may also eventually develop an invasive breast cancer sometime in the future, it is unclear how to assess the risk or determine an appropriate level of intervention.

Dr. Susan Love argues that a stage 0 cancer that does not have the capacity to spread is a very different scenario from a localized breast cancer that does. The problem is that we are unable to determine between these two critically different outcomes. DCIS does increase breast cancer risk, but the risk is about the same as that of a woman without breast cancer who had a late first pregnancy.[22] Studies reported in the mid-1980s found that autopsies done on women who died from a variety of causes found that between 6 and 16 percent had DCIS.[23] Untreated DCIS *can* lead to the later development of an invasive type of breast cancer, but it does not seem to do so in the majority of cases.[24] Existing studies suggest that 20 to 25 percent of women with untreated low-grade (benign) DCIS will go on to develop invasive cancer up to 25 years after the initial biopsy. Yet most people diagnosed with DCIS receive the same treatment as those diagnosed with early-stage invasive breast cancer—surgery, radiation, and mastectomy.[25] If mastectomies were performed on all of these women, 75 to 80 percent would appear to have been cured even though they would have never gotten invasive breast cancer.[26] While Dr. Love stresses that there are a number of possible treatments, Dr. Welch and colleagues emphasize that treatment is not a cure for a disease that poses no apparent threat.[27]

Of the 67,770 cases of *in situ* breast cancers in 2008, 15 percent will be LCIS. The diagnosis of LCIS is determined on the basis of microscopic analysis, and it is usually diagnosed only after a biopsy is taken to examine some other breast condition (e.g., cysts, abscesses, or benign growths). Although this class of *in situ* breast cancer is now less controversial than is DCIS, there is a similar confusion about its classification as a cancer. LCIS begins in the milk-producing glands, but similar to DCIS it is noninvasive and does not penetrate nearby breast tissue. Unlike DCIS, the abnormal cells do *not* have the capacity to develop into invasive breast cancer in the future, so LCIS does not represent that "gray zone" between normal tissue and cancer cells. There is a general consensus that LCIS is *not* technically a cancer or a pre-cancer. More accurately, it is referred to as lobular neoplasia, a collection of abnormal cells in the milk-producing lobules of the breast.

According to the Stanford University Cancer Center, most doctors do not believe that LCIS itself becomes breast cancer. However, about 25 percent of patients who have LCIS tend to develop breast cancer at some point in their lifetime.[28] LCIS is considered to be a "marker" of increased risk. As with DCIS, it is unknown which women diagnosed with the condition may develop an invasive cancer sometime in the future and which ones may not. Treatment for LCIS focuses on how to reduce future risk. These methods include dietary changes, drug treatments such as hormone therapy, and/or increased medical surveillance for the person's lifetime (e.g., mammograms). Treatment usually does not involve removing abnormal cells through surgery, radiation, or chemotherapy. However, since LCIS is a marker of increased risk, the extreme measure of surgically removing both breasts is considered to be a reasonable treatment option for some women.

The diagnosis and treatment of the stage 0 conditions call into question whose interests are being served. Even though most women with LCIS never get breast cancer, the diagnosis of LCIS puts women at an "increased risk," thereby increasing their lifetime dependence on mammography and other medical interventions. DCIS has even broader implications. DCIS accounts for about one in five cases of breast cancer that are detected by mammography.[29] With the rise in mammography screening, more cases of DCIS will be found, and with more cases of DCIS, the total breast cancer incidence goes up. Since DCIS is stage 0, it appears that more cancers are being found "early." Since DCIS is not a cancer and is not life-threatening, it has a high "cure" rate, thereby giving the impression that early detection "saves lives." Most women diagnosed with DCIS will never develop an invasive breast cancer. Despite evidence to the contrary, Komen writes in its *Understanding Breast Cancer Guide,*

"DCIS *often* develops into invasive cancer" (emphasis added).[30] This statement fuels misunderstanding about this stage o condition. Although the prognosis of DCIS was unknown when it was originally named, the classification of DCIS as a cancer has since become firmly intertwined with a strong dedication to screening mammography.

MEDICAL TECHNOLOGY

The NCI estimates that a woman in the United States has a 1 in 8 chance of developing invasive breast cancer during her lifetime, a risk that was about 1 in 11 in 1975.[31] Approximately 40,460 women and 450 men in the United States were estimated to die from the disease in 2008. These data suggest that breast cancer is on the rise, and is 100 times the mortal threat for women than it is for men. If these statistics are generally correct, then 7 out of 8 women will *not* develop invasive breast cancer. What is different about these women? Although scientists have discovered some of the risk factors associated with breast cancer, they account for only 30 percent of cases. We don't know why some women who are at risk for breast cancer do develop the disease, and why other women at risk do not. Yet breast cancer awareness activities have the same recommendation for all women: "Get tested regularly. It is the best way to lower your risk of dying from breast cancer. Screening tests can find breast cancer early, when it's most treatable."[32] Cast as an "early" detection tool, screening mammography is the touchstone for the best-funded and most-publicized breast cancer awareness programs.[33]

Screening mammography involves compressing the breast between two plates and then applying a small dose of radiation to produce an X-ray image that can reveal benign or malignant abnormalities. Between 1987 and 2000, the percentage of women in the United States over age 40 who reported that they had a mammogram in the previous 2 years increased from 39 to 70 percent. Though mammography has been institutionalized as the best protection against breast cancer, it is not without its own controversy and thorny questions. If seven out of eight women would never have developed breast cancer in the first place, is regular screening really necessary for these women? What does "early" detection mean when it comes to cancer, and is it really possible to find life-threatening breast cancers "early" using this medical technology? What are the risks and benefits of mammography screening for women who would never have developed the disease? Do the benefits outweigh the risks equally for all women? Does it really save lives as claimed?

The scientific debate over screening mammography has been ongoing for three decades. Reports in medical journals as early as 1976 identified major problems with mammography screening, such as insufficient data about its accuracy, benefit, and the long-term effects of radiation exposure.[34] A review of clinical trials on the effects of screening in 2000 and an analysis from the Institute of Medicine (IOM) in 2001 re-ignited and publicized the longstanding debate about the benefits, limitations, and risks of screening mammography.

The Benefits of Mammography

The goal of screening for breast cancer is to decrease the death rate, making mortality reduction mammography's primary benefit. Interventions such as mammography have been studied in randomized controlled trials, which carefully assess the benefits and risks of screening for specific groups of people. In randomized controlled trials, participants are assigned to receive a certain screening procedure, and the frequency and extent of use are predetermined. Then the outcomes of these groups are compared to those of control groups that did not receive the intervention. Seven clinical trials conducted between 1963 and 1982 specifically analyzed the impact of screening mammography on mortality. Only one of these had been conducted in the United States. To evaluate the quality of the trials and the evidence they produced, there have been three systematic reviews (meta-analyses) of these initial studies. The following analyses show reductions in mortality resulting from mammography screening to be quite variable, and fairly modest.

The Cochrane Review was first published in the *Lancet* in 2000 by Gøtzsche and Olsen and was reported in more detail in the *Cochrane Library* in 2001.[35] The researchers did a systematic review of seven major randomized controlled trials of screening mammography that involved over half a million women, and assessed the quality of the studies in terms of agreed-upon standards for well-conducted and reliable research. After identifying no trials with high-quality data, two trials with medium-quality data (Canada and Malmö), three trials with poor-quality data (Göteborg, Stockholm, and Two-County), and two trials (Edinburgh and New York) that were highly flawed, they concluded that there was no reliable evidence to justify mass screening. The two trials that were the most methodologically sound did *not* find a reduction in breast cancer mortality, in contrast to the trials with poor-quality data that did (25 percent after 13 years). One of the quality problems involved misclassifying the cause of death. Radiation treatment for early breast cancers tends to reduce the rate of local recurrence, but it also increases the probability of heart failure. If a woman treated with radiation for breast cancer dies during the follow-up period from a heart attack, did her death result from breast cancer treatment or some other reason? Classifying her death as heart failure and not breast cancer, the researchers would argue, is a misclassification of death that biases the studies in favor of screening.

In 2006, Gøtzsche and Nielsen updated the 2000-2001 Cochrane analysis, getting more of the primary data from the studies where they could, including cause of death and study set-up. They identified seven randomized trials that compared mammography screening with no mammography screening, including six trials from the original investigation. Similar to the earlier findings, the trials that were most sound methodologically found no statistically significant reduction in breast cancer mortality compared to the trials that were methodologically flawed. Four of the trials were *not* adequately randomized, which called into question whether the subjects in the screening group may have been healthier than those in the non-screening group or whether their deaths may have been misclassified in terms of other causes. Yet these were the studies to show a significant reduction in breast cancer mortality (35 to 40 percent). The three trials that were randomized adequately, however, did *not* show a significant mortality reduction. Yet compared to unscreened women the screened women were more likely to be diagnosed and treated. The researchers concluded: "For every 2000 women invited for screening throughout 10 years, one will have her life prolonged and 10 healthy women, who would not have been diagnosed if there had not been screening, will be treated unnecessarily."[36] They concluded that screening decreased the risk of death by about 15 percent for women ages 50 to 69, while increasing the risk of overdiagnosis and overtreatment by about 30 percent.

Corroborating the Cochrane conclusions that mass screening was not warranted, the Humphrey review (2002) concluded that the absolute benefit of mammography screening on mortality was only 16 percent, which was quite similar to the conclusion reached by Gøtzsche and Nielson (15 percent). However, Humphrey and colleagues concluded that biases in the trials could statistically eliminate or even produce that reduction.[37] The 2006 Armstrong review, which included 117 studies in addition to the original trials, focused on the effects of screening on mortality reduction specifically for women between the ages of 40 and 49.[38] This is a crucial age group to consider since the standard protocol has been to begin regular screening at age 40, and screening is far less accurate in this age group. The researchers from this analysis also found a wide range of estimated mortality reduction: 7 to 23 percent. For this age group, they determined a rate of false-positives from 20 to 56 percent and subsequent increases in unnecessary procedures. They conclude that for women age 40 to 49, the risks of screening may outweigh the benefits.

The IOM, an arm of the National Academy of Sciences, in 2001 released a report called *Mammography and Beyond* that reviewed breast cancer detection technologies in development and examined technology development and adoption. The reviewers found that screening technologies had not been adequately assessed in terms of their clinical outcomes, thereby mystifying their potential value. They also acknowledged that given the current lack of understanding about premalignant or pre-invasive breast lesions (e.g., DCIS and LCIS), we should *not* assume that the detection of these conditions would reduce mortality or have any increased benefit for women. As a result, the IOM recommended that *new* screening technologies should depend on clinical evidence of improved outcomes—ideally, a reduction in overall mortality. To this end, the IOM urged the NCI to create a permanent infrastructure for testing the efficacy and clinical effectiveness of new technologies for early cancer detection as they emerge.[39] Unfortunately, the evaluation of emergent technologies does not change anything about the use of the technologies we currently have.

Even after considerable national debate spurred by the Gøtzsche analyses and the subsequent IOM report, the NCI maintained its recommendations in testimony to the U.S. Senate that women over 40 should be screened every 1 to 2 years.[40] Although the analyses to date did not provide unequivocal proof about the benefits of screening, the NCI did not believe this warranted a change in policy. NCI revisited the mammography question in 2005, not through the testing of clinical effectiveness as the IOM stressed but through the use of high-level statistical modeling. The Cancer Intervention and Surveillance Modeling Network (CISNET) used retrospective surveillance data to create statistical models to illustrate past trends and to project future trends related to screening and mortality. CISNET concluded that the population-level decrease in breast cancer mortality rates from 1990 to 2000 would not have occurred without a sizeable contribution from mammography.[41] The CISNET results fortified a long-held position of the American Cancer Society and a number of breast cancer organizations that screening is the best protection against dying from breast cancer. NCI stated that the CISNET models are "*not* designed for use by or for cancer patients or clinicians seeking treatment guidance for individual cases" (emphasis added). Statistical modeling for assessing the risks and benefits of screening is quite different from using clinical trials that involve real people in comparison groups who are observed over a period of time.

What does all of this information tell us about the benefits of mammography for actual women? A message from NCI's CancerMail states that "clinical trials are the best way to directly compare the benefits and risks of screening tests."[42] This statement aligns with the position of the World Health Organization (WHO), which developed guidelines in 1968 for evaluating clinical trials of cancer screening technologies. The WHO states that (a) the disorder screened should be an important cause of morbidity (an incidence of ill health), disability, or mortality; (b) the screening tool must be available and acceptable to the target population and that population's physicians; (c) screening should include appropriate follow-up of individuals with a positive result; (d) the screening tool must have acceptable performance characteristics; and (e) the tool should provide a net benefit to the target population. Breast cancer incidence and mortality are high enough to warrant systematic and effective screening, but beyond this, screening mammography falls short. Mammography has been widely promoted despite ongoing scientific and medical controversy. Performance characteristics demonstrate high rates of false-positives, false-negatives, overdiagnosis, and overtreatment, calling mammography's net benefit into question.

Age and menopausal status are critical factors. Studies consistently indicate that mammography screening, if beneficial at all, is *more* beneficial for women ages 50 and 70, and there are few studies of women over age 70.[43] For women over age 50, studies have shown that the average mortality reduction of about 15 to 20 percent (ranging from 0 to 37 percent), with an absolute mortality benefit of 0.05 percent and 10 times the risk of over-diagnosis and overtreatment. For women over age 50 the reduction in mortality is quite small, and individual women cannot know whether they will be part of the smaller percentage of women whose lives are extended or the larger percentage of women whose lives are not.

The American College of Physicians in 2007 moved away from recommending universal screening for women aged 40 to 49 and instead recommended that women make an informed decision after learning about the benefits and harms of mammography.[44] In January 2009, one of the researchers from the Cochrane review stated unequivocally in the *British Medical Journal*, "there is no reliable evidence that screening decreases total mortality, although half a million women participated in the screening trials."[45] On November 19th 2009 the United States Preventative Task Force also reversed screening guidelines. Instead of beginning mammograms at age 40, they recommended starting mammograms at age 50—every two years, instead of annually. They emphasized that these guidelines were aimed at reducing harm from overtreatment.[46] Still, the American Cancer Society website states, "Most doctors feel that early detection tests for breast cancer save many thousands of lives each year, and that many more lives could be saved if even more women and their health care providers took advantage of these tests."[47]

And despite his early statement admitting the over-promise of screening, Dr. Otis Brawley of the American Cancer Society also reversed his position after the task force released the new guidelines. He said: "As someone who has long been a critic of those overstating the benefits of screening, I use these words advisedly: this is one screening test I recommend unequivocally, and would recommend to any woman 40 and over, be she a patient, a stranger, or a family member."[48]

Adding to the confusion about mammography's specific role in reducing mortality are the spurious correlations between the general rise in mammography screening (stated previously) and a general reduction in mortality rates (the number of women per 100,000 women in the United States who die of breast cancer each year). The death rate is standardized to accommodate increases in population size and age, so it is useful in showing change over time. According to the NCI, the decrease in the breast cancer mortality rate has been about 1.8 percent each year from 1989 to 1996.[49] This decline was 2 years after the use of mammography started to rise rapidly. Between 1990 and 2005, death rates decreased 27 percent over 15 years and the decline in mortality was greater for white women than for African American women.[50] Improvements in treatment and early detection are credited for the decline. However, the magnitude of breast cancer mortality is reflected in the actual number of deaths, which has consistently been about 40,000 per year. Significantly, the death rates do not include treatment-related deaths.

The Risks of Mammography

Given the uncertainty over mammography's benefit for women, risk analysis becomes more important. Mammograms frequently provide insufficient information to reach clear conclusions about the presence of tumors, and suspicious areas on a mammogram may or may not indicate cancer. The IOM reported that 75 percent of all positive mammograms, upon biopsy, were "false-positives" (i.e., did *not* show the presence of cancer).[51] The risk of having a false-positive during routine yearly screening is about 10 percent, and according to a study published in the *Journal of the National Cancer Institute*, by the time a woman has had 10 mammograms, she will have a 50 percent chance of being told her results are abnormal.[52] The high rate of false-positives means that the biopsies were not necessary for the majority of women who had them. If the biopsy sample does not contain enough tissue to make a definite diagnosis, women are then subjected to multiple biopsies. These procedures are invasive, anxiety-producing, and costly. The cost of a breast biopsy can range from approximately $1,000 to $5,000, depending on the type of biopsy, the equipment used, and the facility.[53] Many health maintenance plans require referrals prior to the procedure, and the cost may be prohibitive for the 23 million women (nearly one in five) in the United States who have no health insurance.[54]

Second, mammograms on average miss 25 to 40 percent of tumors that actually *are* cancerous.[55] These are called "false-negatives." There are several reasons why mammograms miss these cancers, including the ability of the X-ray to clearly capture the image, the lack of certainty about how to interpret "suspicious" areas on the image, differences in the ability of radiologists to assess the image accurately, and the rate of tumor growth. Mammograms are better able to "see" through fatty breast tissue than through dense breast tissue, increasing the accuracy of the image for women with more fatty tissue. Since premenopausal women generally have denser breasts, mammograms are less accurate for these women than for postmenopausal women. However, mammograms are very good at seeing calcium deposits even in dense breasts. Calcium deposits (microcalcifications) are very common in women, especially as they age, are common in benign breast conditions, and may also form around dead cells in DCIS and LCIS. For these reasons, it is difficult to interpret what their presence on a mammogram indicates. DCIS, for example, is almost always diagnosed when a mammogram shows calcium deposits and a subsequent biopsy shows cell irregularities (abnormal hyperplasia). Such irregularities fall into that gray zone between normal tissue and invasive cancer, as discussed earlier, making this condition difficult to diagnose. However, for invasive breast cancers, only certain types of microcalcifications are associated with higher-grade tumors, and even these are not independent prognostic factors.[56]

Also, radiologists have different levels of experience and criteria for assessing mammograms. A study published in the *Journal of the National Cancer Institute* reported that radiologists' ability to accurately read diagnostic mammograms varies from

27 to 100 percent, with radiologists who work at academic medical centers more likely to be accurate.[57] A final difficulty is that cancers grow at different rates. A high rate of growth, when more than 6 to 10 percent of the cells are making new cells, may help to predict how aggressive a cancer is. When it comes to detection, slow-growing tumors are simply around longer and are therefore easier to catch. Faster-growing, more life-threatening tumors are more likely to appear between screenings, having been missed by the earlier mammogram.[58]

Third, the detection of abnormal tissue that will never become symptomatic is a form of "overdiagnosis" that contributes to the inflation of incidence statistics. The stage 0 *in situ* conditions currently represent about 23 percent of breast cancer diagnoses each year, and the incidence rates for these types have been on the rise. The diagnosis of DCIS has increased from 1 to 2 percent of all breast cancers 20 years ago to 17 percent in 1997 and 23 percent in 2005. According to an article in the *Journal of the American Medical Association*, the more than 23,000 cases of DCIS diagnosed in 1992 were 200 percent higher than might be expected from rates in 1983, and from trends between 1973 and 1983.[59] By 2008, that number more than doubled again to over 57,000 cases. Until the 1980s, when mammography use expanded widely, DCIS was rarely found because DCIS is not found with a clinical breast examination; DCIS is almost always detected by mammograms. Screening mammography is largely responsible for the ever-increasing diagnoses of stage 0 breast cancers, the types that are not *technically* breast cancers at all.

Fourth, overdiagnosis leads to overtreatment, resulting in 30 percent more surgery, 20 percent more mastectomies, and more use of radiotherapy.[60] Seventy percent of DCIS lesions remain harmless for a lifetime, and the long-term survival rate is nearly 100 percent regardless of treatment. There is also research showing that spontaneous regression of breast cancer may be more common than people think.[61] Yet DCIS is diagnosed more frequently and treated more aggressively in the United States than anywhere else in the world. In 2002, 26 percent of DCIS patients were treated with mastectomy. Other treatments included lumpectomy, radiation, chemotherapy, and hormone therapy such as tamoxifen. If an abnormality does not cause symptoms and is not likely to progress to invasive cancer, then the risks associated with surgery, radiation damage, ongoing radiation from regular mammography, anxiety about risk, side effects of systemic therapy, and increased medical costs may far outweigh the benefits of treatment.[62]

Fifth, is it possible that increased mammography actually causes more breast cancer? A fundamental assumption to screening programs is that early detection will lead to an eventual decline in invasive breast cancers in the future. A Scandinavian study published in 2004 found no corresponding long-term reduction in the rate of women diagnosed with breast cancer.[63] Instead, after mammography screening was introduced in Norway for women aged 50 to 69 years, the incidence of breast cancer increased by 54 percent. Similarly, after mammography screening began in Sweden in 1987 breast cancer incidence increased by 45 percent. The researchers concluded that "without screening, one third of all invasive breast cancers in the age group 50-69 years would not have been detected in the patients' lifetime."

The U.S. Food and Drug Administration (FDA) acknowledges that the lifetime risk of developing cancer increases with radiation exposure from X-rays. A person who undergoes more X-ray examinations has an accumulated radiation risk. People who receive X-rays at a younger age have a greater risk than those who are older. Women are at a higher lifetime risk than men for developing cancer from radiation after receiving the same exposures at the same ages.[64] According to the FDA, a mammogram is comparable to 3 months of exposure to natural background radiation. An 80-year-old woman who had a mammogram every 2 years from the age of 40 will have been exposed to an additional 5 years of radiation in her lifetime. In a review of 47 scientific articles about mammography, Samuel S. Epstein, MD, Professor Emeritus of Environmental Medicine at the University of Illinois at Chicago School of Public Health, and his colleagues concluded that in addition to false-positives, false-negatives, and overdiagnosis, another danger of mammography screening is the induction and promotion of breast cancer.[65] For women who carry a genetic mutation associated with increased breast cancer risk, studies have found that radiation from mammograms may promote the spread of cancer cells.[66]

Cost/Benefit Analysis

Do the benefits of mammography outweigh the risks? Every diagnosed woman must determine this for herself based on her own situational context. Yet how is a person to make this determination? The questionable status of mammography as the solution to the breast cancer problem has placed the burden of risk assessment on women themselves. How are women to assess the risks when every T-shirt, ad campaign, and pink ribbon comes fully equipped with the unequivocal message that "early detection saves lives"?

Even official medical information amplifies the benefits of mammography while minimizing or omitting the risks. A 2006 survey of the content of information given to women who were invited for mammography screening in six countries concluded that "one-sided propaganda about breast screening...resulted in misconceptions about its effects."[67] The information did not mention the risks of overdiagnosis and overtreatment of healthy women at all. One third of the invitations stated that screening leads to either less invasive surgery or simpler treatment, even though overdiagnosis produces the opposite effect. Half of the invitations mentioned the possibility of pain, a temporary and the least serious harmful effect of screening. Although the researchers produced an evidence-based leaflet that outlined the benefits and risks of screening, a 2009 follow-up showed little change.[68]

Similarly inaccurate or misleading information is used in the screening programs in the United States. The American Cancer Society states:

> Only 2 to 4 mammograms of every 1,000 lead to a diagnosis of cancer. About 10% of women who have a mammogram will require more tests, and the majority will only need an additional mammogram. Don't panic if this happens to you. Only 8% to 10% of those women will need a biopsy, and most (80%) of those biopsies will not be cancer.[69]

Downplaying the inaccuracy of mammograms and unnecessary biopsies solidifies social investment in mammography screening. As Chapter 2 pointed out, the staunch commitment to mammography has a long history tied to National Breast Cancer Awareness Month (NBCAM) and the pink ribbon, which together provide a springboard for public investment in breast cancer as a women's health epidemic. The Komen Affiliate Network is "the nation's largest private funder of community-based breast health education and breast cancer screening and treatment programs," with 130 affiliate organizations.[70] Komen disseminates its central message of early detection through these organizations: "Getting tested regularly is the best way for women to lower their risk of dying from breast cancer. Screening tests can find breast cancer early, when it's most treatable."

Under the category "Quality of Screening Tests," Komen downplays the inaccuracy of mammography, stating "there is no such thing as a perfect screening test with 100 percent sensitivity and 100 percent specificity. There is usually give-and-take between the two." Komen then dismisses the risk of false-positives under the heading "Accuracy of Mammograms," stating: "The most important job of mammography is to find as many early cancers as possible, not to avoid false-positive results. False-positive results may cause unnecessary anxiety. However, this does not outweigh the life-saving value of regular screening."[71] Komen not only disregards the inaccuracy of screening and replaces it with statements that stress survival, but the website's search mechanism produces no material for the terms "overdiagnosis" and "overtreatment."

Balanced information is lacking in pink ribbon culture, but it is possible to establish sound principles for evaluating the costs and benefits of any medical intervention. A number of organizations, including the National Breast Cancer Coalition, the New York State Breast Cancer Support and Education Network, the Breast Cancer Fund, Breast Cancer Action, the Collaborative on Health and the Environment, and numerous other community-based advocacy organizations have committed to evidence-based assessments of scientific and medical information. The National Breast Cancer Coalition's Project LEAD teaches laypersons to understand biomedical technoscience in ways that enable them to make decisions about breast cancer as well as influence research and policy agendas. The burgeoning environmental breast cancer movement has used scientific research and biomedical knowledge of cancer-causing agents to raise awareness of environmental causes and promote precautionary measures, including removing known toxic agents from everyday products and environments.[72] These mobilizations, which will be discussed in the concluding chapter, are gaining momentum despite pressure from the cancer industry and pink ribbon culture to submit to medicalization and avoid scientific controversies.

Screening Programs and the Makers of the Machines

By 2005, the percentage of women getting regular mammograms dropped slightly from 70 to 66 percent, according to estimates from the National Health Interview Survey.[73] The reason for the decline could be related to increasing public awareness about the ongoing mammography controversy. Certainly, statements from the American College of Physicians, the IOM, and the National Breast Cancer Coalition were able to create some functional awareness about mammography's limitations. Still, screening creates customers, jobs, research agendas, revenues, and profits. Those who profit the most from screening programs have a vested interest in maintaining the message that "early detection" through mammography screening "is the key." In particular, the companies that develop and manufacture imaging technology have a lot to lose if women stop having regular mammograms.

According to the NCI, screening mammograms generally cost between $50 and $150.[74] This amount does not take into account the variation in price depending upon what insurance companies are willing to pay, who has coverage, the kind of coverage, and the added costs of mammogram-related services. Many states, for example, require health insurance companies to pay for regular mammograms for women over age 40. The insurance company then negotiates this coverage with providers and determines the deductibles that the insured person must pay.[75] Many women over the years have told me that their insurance companies charged them upwards of $500, and sometimes thousands of dollars, for a mammogram they thought would be fully covered. Part of the reason is that the cost for a single screening may also include charges for outpatient hospital services, radiologist fees, ultrasounds, follow-up mammograms, and biopsies due to the high rate of false-positives. According to the 2000 Census, there are about 53 million women in the United States between the ages of 40 and 75.[76] If 66 percent of the women in this age group have an average-priced ($150) mammogram every 2 years, the United States will be spending a minimum of $2.62 billion annually on diagnostic screening alone. Since the costs vary upwards, the number is probably much higher.

For uninsured women, compliance with screening protocols requires out-of-pocket payment or enrollment in a program that offers low-cost or free mammograms, and there are many of these programs across the country. Still, the prices vary. The mobile mammography van in my community submits claims for women who have insurance with Blue Cross Blue Shield of Texas but charges $219.80 at the time of service to those without insurance. They accept cash, check, Visa, or MasterCard. Another organization charges uninsured and underinsured women between $65 and $70 for a mammogram. In addition to costs to the uninsured medical consumer, how much does it cost each year for an organization to run a mobile mammography unit, and how is it funded? A community-based organization that provided 1,300 free mammograms and 700 low-cost ($65 to $70) mammograms in 2008 paid not only for a portion of the total mammograms, but also for equipment and maintenance, supplies, technicians, radiologists, administration of services, accreditation and inspections, liability insurance, and advertising. Mobile units also require drivers, fuel, and maintenance. Typical operating costs for one mobile screening program totaled about $400,000 per year. To fund the program, the organization relied on grants from the American Cancer Society and large-scale breast cancer organizations with a vested interest in the mammography screening project, as well as other funding agencies. The $2.62 billion spent per year on screening just got bigger, and the proliferation of screening as the only public health strategy to deal with breast cancer is now virtually guaranteed in communities across the country.

The investment in screening also exists at the federal level. The Centers for Disease Control and Prevention administers 68 state, tribal, and territorial programs that collectively represent the National Breast and Cervical Cancer Early Detection Program (NBCCEDP).[77] Federal guidelines establish an eligibility baseline for breast screening of uninsured and underinsured women between the ages of 40 and 64 at or below 250 percent of the federal poverty level. From 1991 through 2002, 1.2 million women received over 2 million mammograms through the program, and less than 1 percent (9,956) were diagnosed with breast cancer. Of these, 73 percent were diagnosed with an invasive breast cancer at stages 1 or 2.[78] Until Congress passed the Breast and Cervical Cancer Prevention and Treatment Act in 2000, which gives states the option to offer women in the program access to treatment through Medicaid, women who were diagnosed through the program had to find their own means for treatment. To date, every state has approved the Medicaid option, and Congress extended it to American Indians and Alaska Natives in 2001. From 2003 through 2007, NBCCEDP provided 1.8 million mammograms and reported a detection rate of 8.4 invasive or *in situ* breast cancers for every 1,000 women screened (less than 1 percent). A cost analysis of nine participating programs found that the median total cost of screening services to women was $555 per woman served.[79]

If mammography saves enough lives, then the investment may be worth it; certainly, it is worth it for women who were diagnosed with an invasive breast cancer and then given high-quality, effective treatment that staved off their illness and improved their quality of life. Given the limitations and dangers of mammography described earlier, the unquestioned investment in screening at local, state, and national levels is dubious. Yet the widespread investment in screening has guaranteed that those who develop and manufacture imaging technology are at the center of a huge profit-making endeavor.

General Electric introduced the industry's first dedicated breast imaging system in 1966. From that initial foray, GE created a new and successful profit center in medical technology. A 2007 article in *Medical Product Outsourcing* (MPO) magazine reported that revenues from the medical imaging equipment industry grew from about $3 billion in 1997 to over $9 billion 10 years later.[80] Healthcare research analysts predict that the market for medical imaging equipment (not including services) is expected to thrive at a 7.6 percent compound annual growth rate. A vice president for Siemens Medical Solutions said that one of the reasons for the market's continued growth is that imaging technology has been "growing by leaps and bounds in almost direct proportion to advances in the computer industry." These technological advances have led to improvements in some aspects of medical imaging, including resolution, processing speed, data storage and retrieval, and even smaller equipment. More importantly, these changes have impelled a major shift in research and development, with a strong focus on the conversion from film mammography (analog) to digital imaging systems that are better able to use computer-based platforms.

Digital mammography is more efficient and convenient than analog. However, when comparing diagnostic accuracy, a clinical study from the American College of Radiology Imaging Network[81] reported that digital mammography did *not* perform better than film for the overall population of participants—nor did it perform better for women over age 50, women who were postmenopausal (the group that represents more than 75 percent of the population diagnosed with breast cancer), or women who did not have dense breast tissue. Digital mammography did perform better for younger women, making the new technology potentially useful for diagnosing high-risk, younger women with dense breast tissue. Even though the outcome data do not adequately support a widespread move to the more expensive digital systems, the technological imperative (along with profits) continues to fuel the system.

GE spent $100 million over 10 years on research and development for digital detection equipment alone.[82] By 2000, GE introduced the world's first full-field digital mammography system, Senographe, which was on display at the 91st annual meeting of the Radiological Society of North America. Since Senographe's introduction, more than 1,500 of the GE systems have been installed worldwide. By 2005, GE announced three new advanced imaging technologies to augment the Senographe system.[83] Today, 8 percent of the 10,000 breast cancer screening centers in the United States use digital systems, up from 6 percent in 2007. As a market leader in digital mammography, GE's technology infrastructure generated a 14 percent increase ($5.1 billion) in revenue for the corporation in 2007. Diagnostic imaging is so lucrative that GE even expects its global healthcare business of $9 billion to offset weaknesses due to the current economic downturn in the United States.

Digital imaging units can cost from $300,000 to $500,000, so conversion to digital mammography is an expensive endeavor.

Even though more screening centers are converting to digital systems, there were still only 2,500 digital systems in the United States in 2007, compared to about 13,000 film-based systems. Some of these were leased. A community-based organization in New York, Breast Cancer Help, Inc., had a 63-month lease for the new GE system and began making lease payments in excess of $7,000 per month.[84] The systems are cost-prohibitive for many screening centers. However, costs could come down. The FDA recently approved the Fuji digital mammography system for sale in the United States. Already the most widely used system internationally, the Fuji system (about $200,000) is roughly half the cost of GE's digital mammography equipment.[85] GE may have a run for its money. Still, GE Healthcare is a $17 billion division of GE that sells healthcare products and services worldwide to hospitals, medical facilities, pharmaceutical and biotechnology companies, and the life science research market. With active marketing campaigns, relationships with major breast cancer organizations, and vertical and horizontal leveraging across a constellation of industries from mass media to aviation to utilities to health, GE is likely to have the resources to beat the competition with flying colors.

BIG PHARMA

As the technological imperative thrusts forward, a group of about 15 pharmaceutical companies known as "Big Pharma" lead the pack in developing new medications and new ways to use drugs. With combined global sales in the trillions of dollars,[86] Big Pharma constitutes one of the most powerful and profitable industries in the world, and prescription drugs are the foundation of the industry's profits. The United States spent $216.7 billion for prescription drugs in 2006, which was 5 times the $40.3 billion spent in 1990 and 18 times the $12 billion spent in 1980.[87] The U.S. Department of Health and Human Services projects that prescription drug spending in the United States will increase to $515.7 billion in 2017, a 138 percent increase in 11 years.[88] In 2007, the top 25 pharmacy benefit management companies dispensed over 3.6 billion prescriptions.[89] Cancer drugs are the fastest-growing and best-selling class of drugs in this rapidly expanding market, and every major drug company is investing heavily in oncology-related research and development. Sales of oncology drugs grew from under $5 billion in 1998 to over $19 billion by 2008, and analysts predict that oncology drug costs will rise 20 percent each year for the next 5 years. Oncology drugs represent the largest share of the global drug market, and sales are projected to grow at a compounded annual rate of 12 to 15 percent, reaching $75 to $80 billion by 2012.[90]

Since 2003, Pfizer increased the number of oncology research and development projects by 400 percent and now dedicates 22 percent of its total budget to oncology. The company has 22 oncology compounds in a total of 232 ongoing, planned, or sponsored oncology clinical studies.[91] Sales of oncology and nausea drugs for GlaxoSmithKline (GSK), the second largest

U.S. pharmaceutical company, represented 2 percent ($814 million) of the company's total drug sales in 2008.[92] GSK's drug Tykerb for advanced breast cancer was approved for use in the United States in 2007 and in Europe in 2008, with patents expiring in 2020 and 2023, respectively. Though these were a smaller share of total revenues, GSK's annual report states, "Oncology is an important investment area for GSK and 2008 has seen its late stage pipeline flourish."[93] To this end, the company created an integrated oncology unit to identify and develop new drugs. To create them faster and cheaper, GSK reorganized its research and development infrastructure so that about half of the new drugs would come from outside partners instead of internal development efforts.

New drug markets and more expensive drugs generate higher profits for the industry and help to maintain the market leverage of the biggest of Big Pharma. Pfizer and GSK lead the industry, followed closely by AstraZeneca, which relied on oncology drugs for 12 percent of its revenue in 2007. AstraZeneca's drug Nolvadex (tamoxifen) has been a standard therapy for premenopausal women with early-stage breast cancer or certain types of metastatic breast cancer for the past 30 years. First obtaining FDA approval in 1986, tamoxifen enjoyed six different FDA approvals through 2000, expanding its applications every time. Because patent life can be extended with the approval of new indications, companies are constantly searching for new disease classifications to treat with old drugs. By 2001, global sales of tamoxifen reached over $1 billion. Following the drug's patent expiration in 2002, less expensive generic options reduced its market share. This was not too much of a problem for AstraZeneca because the company had already developed and had been widely distributing Arimidex (anastrozole), a treatment drug for postmenopausal women. Since the risk of breast cancer is highest after menopause, Arimidex would potentially reach a greater number of women diagnosed with breast cancer. Arimidex was also successful in expanding its applications with successive FDA approvals.

Marketing life-cycle management programs for products such as AstraZeneca's hormone-based cancer treatments enable pharmaceutical companies to leverage their investment in a drug within the time frame that patent protection is available. Arimidex had first obtained FDA approval in 1995 to treat postmenopausal women with advanced breast cancer whose disease had progressed after treatment with tamoxifen. In 2000, the FDA approved the same drug for a second group—first-line treatment of postmenopausal women with locally advanced or metastatic breast cancer in which the hormone receptors were either positive or unknown. (In hormone receptor–positive breast cancers, either estrogen or progesterone fuels tumor growth. These types of breast cancers may respond to treatments that suppress the actions of hormones in the body.) Then the drug obtained preliminary approval in 2002 and final approval in 2005 for a third group—postsurgical treatment of postmenopausal women with hormone receptor–positive early breast cancer. With each new FDA approval, AstraZeneca expanded its sales to a broader market of diagnosed women. By 2007, worldwide sales of Arimidex totaled $1.7 billion. When the patent was due to expire in December 2009, the FDA granted an additional 6-month period of exclusivity.[94] By expanding the drug's applications throughout its patent life, AstraZeneca maximized the drug's commercial potential.

Generic competition at the end of a successful drug's patent life is a threat to company profits. Big Pharma leverages this threat by using existing compounds from previously patented drugs to develop new applications, and therefore new patents. These drugs, called "me-too" drugs, are classified as being better than the previously patented drugs, though they are ostensibly used for the same purposes. Marcia Angell, of the Department of Social Medicine at Harvard Medical School, and former editor of the *New England Journal of Medicine*, found that only 14 percent of the FDA's newly approved drugs between 1998 and 2004 were actually new chemical compounds.[95] Likewise, AstraZeneca's hormone-based drug Faslodex (fulvestrant) has the same application as Arimidex—to treat postmenopausal women with metastatic breast cancer who have hormone receptor–positive tumors and who experienced disease progression after anti-estrogen therapies. Faslodex obtained FDA approval in 2002, well in advance of Arimidex's patent expiration. Although the first patent for Faslodex expired in December 2007, a later patent is not set to expire until January 2021. The overlap in patent protection between the two drugs gives continuity to the company's target market while protecting AstraZeneca from generic competition.[96]

In addition to the development of new types of cancer drugs to accommodate a variety of treatment protocols, the costs of cancer drugs are on the rise. Fifteen years ago, the drug Taxol (paclitaxel) from Bristol-Myers was the only commonly used cancer drug that cost over $2,500 per month. But according to a commentary published in the *Journal of the National Cancer Institute*, more than 90 percent of cancer drugs approved in the United States since 2005 cost over $20,000 for a 12-week course of treatment.[97] Genentech's Avastin (bevacizumab), Eli Lilly's Erbitux (cetuximab), and Novartis' Gleevec (imatinib), which are all widely used, cost more than $10,000 per month.[98] Health economists are concerned that the prices of cancer drugs appear to be rising faster than the health benefits associated with them.[99] The competition for new drugs as key weapons in the war against breast cancer carries on often without adequate information about their long-term risks and benefits.

Two key examples relevant to breast cancer involve high-dose chemotherapy and HRT. During the past two decades, approximately 16,000 patients in the United States have undergone high-dose chemotherapy with bone marrow transplant or stem cell support. In clinical trials, the side effects included severe infections, hearing loss, nerve and heart damage, and even death. In its early years, 15 to 20 percent of the patients died from the treatment.[100] In 1999, the results of five randomized trials on high-dose chemotherapy in breast cancer patients were presented at the annual meeting of the American Society of Clinical Oncology. One of these studies was invalidated because it was discovered that the researchers falsified the data.[101] The four remaining studies found that high-dose chemotherapy was no more effective than standard chemotherapy at reducing mortality.[102] Overstating the benefits and concealing the risks in clinical trials parallels the industry's approach to highly profitable drugs.

Wyeth Pharmaceutical's deception about the benefits of HRT is a stark example of the pharmaceutical industry's fraudulent practices in pursuit of profits. HRT is the use of synthetic hormones to "replace" the estrogen and/or progesterone that naturally declines when women approach menopause. Wyeth developed two HRT drugs: Premarin, an estrogen-only pill, and Prempro, a combination estrogen–progestin pill. The drugs received FDA approval to treat menopause and prevent osteoporosis, and in 2002 about 38 percent of postmenopausal women in the United States used some type of HRT. There were 1.62 million prescriptions for Prempro and 3.45 million prescriptions for Premarin that year. Beyond FDA-approved applications, Wyeth heavily promoted HRT for off-label applications, including prevention of heart disease and stroke, while downplaying cancer risks.[103]

Despite the widespread use of HRT drugs, the benefits and risks associated with them had been in question for some time. In 1993, NIH started a clinical trial to examine the effects of longer-term HRT use. From 1993 to 1998, the Women's Health Initiative (WHI) enrolled more than 16,000 women ages 50 and 79 to participate in the 8-year study. Half of the women were randomly assigned to a test group that would receive HRT, and the other half were randomly assigned to a control group that would receive a placebo. While the WHI clinical trial was being implemented, other researchers were publishing conflicting findings from observational studies. The *New England Journal of Medicine* published an article in 1995 from the Nurses' Health Study, which concluded that 5 or more years of HRT was associated with a 46 percent *increase* in breast cancer risk.[104] Two weeks later, the *Journal of the American Medical Association* published an article with opposite results, stating that HRT did not appear to be associated with an increased risk of breast cancer.[105]

With the findings from the WHI study still years away, confusion about the risks and benefits associated with HRT continued in the scientific medical community, leaving doctors and patients to fend for themselves. When asked how to make sense of the conflicting data about HRT and breast cancer, Dr. Leon Speroff, professor of obstetrics and gynecology at Oregon Health Sciences University School of Medicine, said on WebMD: "In my opinion, in the absence of studies, in the absence of data, there is no right or wrong answer."[106] This kind of lax sentiment prevailed. Instead of stopping the production and distribution of HRT drugs until the WHI trial had been completed, Premarin and Prempro continued to be some of the most widely prescribed drugs, and Wyeth marketed them aggressively for off-label applications. By 2002, there was conclusive evidence that HRT's health risks far exceeded its benefits. NIH halted the WHI study with 3 years to go because the women in the test group had significant increases in breast cancer, heart attacks, strokes, and blood clots.[107] The study was simply too dangerous to continue, and it unequivocally confirmed what had been a growing but too often ignored body of evidence.

After information about the WHI trial was released and the news media ran the story, sales of Prempro and Premarin plummeted.[108] With the immediate drop in HRT use, breast cancer incidence rates in the United States also dropped.[109] In the midst of the public controversy, a Wyeth spokesperson upheld support for the company's product, stating: "We believe in the value of hormone replacement therapy…and will continue to support the franchise in the marketplace."[110] By 2007, Wyeth faced over 5,000 lawsuits in federal and state courts on behalf of approximately 8,400 women for injuries related to the HRT drugs. Sales representative Brett Hendricks provided testimony regarding his 21-year career with Wyeth: "That's how we were trained…To offset any bad publicity, we would redirect and emphasize the benefits of the product and say the benefits far outweighed any problems that might be out there."[111] Fifty-seven million prescriptions for HRT continue to be filled in the United States,[112] and in 2008 Wyeth announced that it was already developing a new HRT variation, named Aprela.[113]

INDUSTRY TIES TO ADVOCACY

The leaders of cancer industry use pink ribbon culture and its roots in breast cancer advocacy to maintain a strong competitive edge in the cancer marketplace. As discussed in previous chapters, the rise in breast cancer publicity since the early 1990s fostered greater public awareness of the illness (couched as fear and risk) and a mandate for prevention and research (counterpoised as hope and action). Every October, NBCAM serves as the official platform for pink ribbon culture to advertise treatment, promote early detection, encourage fundraising, and promise eventual disease eradication. Since the pink platform now extends beyond October and saturates the fabric of American life year-round, the industry has greater incentive to promote certain disease classifications along with new and improved medical technologies and pharmaceuticals that will guarantee an expanding array of products and services for the industry's most valued customers—women at risk for, or diagnosed with, breast cancer. To affect how their customers think about breast cancer, industry leaders use savvy marketing campaigns and tactical relationships with key breast cancer organizations, such as branding and cause-marketing strategies.

The commitment to early detection vis-à-vis mammography as the only public health approach to breast cancer began with the establishment of NBCAM in 1985. Zeneca, the company that sponsored NBCAM through the American Cancer Society, was a subsidiary of one of the world's largest multinational chemical corporations, Imperial Chemical Industries. As part of ICI, Zeneca manufactured and marketed tamoxifen, one of the most commonly prescribed cancer treatment drugs. In 1997 Zeneca received 49 percent of its profits from the sale of pesticides and other industrial chemicals (some of which contribute to cancer), 49 percent from pharmaceutical sales, and the remaining 2 percent from healthcare services, which included

II cancer treatment centers. Maren Klawiter explains: "Zeneca pharmaceuticals not only bankrolls and controls the publicity for NBCAM's breast cancer early detection campaigns, but they also, through their parent company ICI, manufacture the pesticides and insecticides that contribute to causing it."[114] In 1999, Zeneca improved its image when it merged with Swedish pharmaceutical company Astra AB to form AstraZeneca and then sold its agricultural chemicals company in 2000 in response to pressure from activists. In addition to the development and sale of oncology drugs, the corporation continues to play a key role in NBCAM through its Healthcare Foundation.

The range of promotional materials that industry leaders use to sway public opinion about breast cancer and promote very specific health behaviors is far-ranging, from websites to press releases, to participation or sponsorship of pink ribbon events, to direct-to-consumer advertising, to logos on pink merchandise. The NBCAM website, sponsored by AstraZeneca, explains how to promote early detection and offers sample media materials, along with tips for getting media attention. NBCAM's website reports over 1 million visits per year.[115] The media materials available for download include a sample press release, sample public service announcements, and a sample proclamation urging "all women and their families in {locality, city, or state} to get the facts about mammography." The website's sample press release offers "the facts" written as a quotation from an "expert":

If all women age 40 and older took advantage of early detection methods—mammography plus clinical breast exam—

breast cancer death rates would drop much further, up to 30 percent," says {insert name and affiliation of local expert}.[116]

The information in the sample press exaggerates the benefits, omits the risks, and encourages individuals to propagate the mythology about mammography without question.

Corporations in the breast cancer industry spend billions of dollars each year to promote early detection while marketing their own revenue-producing solutions to the epidemic. While profiting each year from the imaging technology used to diagnose breast cancer, GE boasts:

> Consumers can make a difference in the fight against breast cancer thanks to the new GE Breast Cancer Awareness cordless phone from Thomson. The company will support research and education for early detection by donating a percentage of the net sales of the phone to the National Breast Cancer Foundation. The product will feature the official pink ribbon memorializing Breast Cancer victims and survivors alike, and the GE brand logo has been changed to a matching pink color.[117]

Echoing NBCAM and the rhetoric of consumer-based agency, GE aligns with pink ribbon culture and softens its public image by offering to memorialize the diagnosed by pinking its logo.

GE has a history of overstatement when it comes to advertising. In the 1990s, GE ran televised advertisements that claimed "a remarkable 91 percent cure rate" for its analog (film) mammography technology. Although the ads supported the general message that "early detection saves lives," the quoted cure rate was actually a 5-year survival rate for early-stage breast cancer. Maryann Napoli of the Center for Medical Consumers argued that being alive in the fifth year after one's diagnosis is not equivalent to a cure that would return a person to a normal life span.[118] GE's ads for the next generation of imaging, full-field digital mammography, claimed that Senographe would "change breast care forever."

Drug companies also spend billions of dollars each year on direct-to-consumer advertising (DTCA) to persuade people to "ask your doctor about [fill in the blank]." In 2008, DTCA for prescription products on television, radio, magazines and newspapers, and outdoor advertising venues totaled $4.4 billion, a 500 percent increase in spending since 1996.[119] Advertising is all about the manipulation of emotion, getting consumers to feel a particular way that will connect them with a product, service, company, or cause. Consumers then put pressure on doctors to use those drugs, often the newer and more expensive ones.

Just as GE pinks its logo to align with pink ribbon culture, ads for cancer drugs use the breast cancer brand to draw on the culture's common themes. Ads for Arimidex feature women in pink boxing gloves ready to face their opponent with feminine style and power. AstraZeneca's full-page ad includes "questions you may want to ask" your doctor. Readers are advised to "Tear out this page. You may find it helpful when talking with your doctor at your next appointment."[120] An ad for Novartis Pharmaceutical's product Femara (letrozole) states: "You had breast cancer. You had Tamoxifen. Now what?... Is there anything more you can do to increase your chances of staying cancer free?" These ads use the themes of the breast cancer brand (fear, hope, and goodness) to promote an emotional connection with the she-ro, the medical consumer who must individually, optimistically, and proactively do all she can to win her personal battle. Consistently drawing on the breast cancer brand and the pink ribbon culture, it enables the industry to forge connections with medical consumers and supply the weapons of choice in the war against breast cancer.

In addition to pink-inspired advertising and corporate philanthropy, the industry forges reciprocal relationships with key players in pink ribbon culture. In addition to its central role in NBCAM, for example, AstraZeneca is closely tied to Komen for the Cure. Although the drug company is not listed as an official corporate sponsor or donor, Komen receives a portion of its operating funds from each of its 122 affiliates, which receive their contributions from individual and corporate donors. In the first 6 months of 2008, AstraZeneca's financial reports listed $97,000 in contributions to several Komen affiliates for general support, fundraisers, and an awareness event for legislators related to their local Komen races. Since Komen for the Cure's financial reports provide only summary financial information for its affiliates, AstraZeneca's financial support is embedded within the $171.3 million in total net revenue for affiliates in 2007.

AstraZeneca's relationship with Komen goes beyond contributions. After AstraZencea received a Friend in the Fight Award from Komen in 2003, the corporation then launched a global breast cancer awareness campaign, "Redefining Hope and Beauty," in 2004 to spread the NBCAM (and Komen's) message internationally.[121]

Similarly, Bristol-Meyers Squibb—in addition to manufacturing and marketing chemotherapy drugs—was a corporate sponsor for the Komen 2008 National Race for the Cure. Its Lawrenceville, New Jersey, facility has hosted the race each October since 2003, raising over $1 million annually.[122] In 2008, Komen partnered with the Young Survival Coalition and Living Beyond Breast Cancer to host the only international conference addressing the concerns of young breast cancer survivors. The goal of this conference is to enable young women with breast cancer and their loved ones to make informed choices with the most up-to-the minute and age-appropriate information about their treatment and well-being. It is "also part of Komen's mission to raise awareness and promote engagement in the breast cancer cause among young women, a powerful generation of advocates." In addition to the Avon Foundation, key sponsors and benefactors include Big Pharma: Bristol-Myers Squibb, Genentech, Novartis, Allergan, GSK, Merck, Pfizer, Wyeth, and AstraZeneca.[123] In collaboration with breast cancer advocacy organizations whose missions aim at supporting and empowering women to make informed choices, these corporations are able to gain access to, and credibility with, members of their key market.

The idea that users of health services should be able to make informed decisions about their medical choices seemingly places control in the hands of patients and advocates. In reality, the medical system, the breast cancer industry, and pink ribbon culture work together to control the information women need when making their choices, while defining the options available to them. The industry that benefits from the increased use of mammography and pharmaceuticals is at the core of what has become pink ribbon culture.

NOTES

1. K. Garrison, "The Personal is Rhetorical: War, Protest, and Peace in Breast Cancer Narratives," *Disability Studies Quarterly* 27, no. 4 (Fall 2007).

2. "National Cancer Act of 1971," National Cancer Institute. http://www.cancer.gov/aboutnci/national-cancer-act-1971/allpages#eec17f26-dbc4-4e77-92fe-1229f6c2d5a8.

3. M. Klawiter, "Breast Cancer in Two Regimes: The Impact of Social Movements on Illness Experience," *Sociology of Health & Illness* 26 (September 2004): 845-74.

4. E. J. Feuer & L.-M. Wun, "How Much of the Recent Rise in Breast Cancer Incidence Can Be Explained by Increases in Mammography Utilization? A Dynamic Population Model Approach," *American Journal of Epidemiology* 136, no. 12 (1992): 1423-36.

5. M. Mayer, *After Breast Cancer: Answers to the Questions You're Afraid to Ask* (Cambridge: O'Reilly, 2003), 34. See also M. Mayer, *Advanced Breast Cancer: A Guide to Living with Metastatic Disease* (Sebastopol, CA: O'Reilly, 1998).

6. American Cancer Society, *Cancer Facts and Figures 2008* (Atlanta: American Cancer Society, 2008).

7. C. Borger et al., "Health Spending Projections Through 2015: Changes on the Horizon," *Health Affairs Web Exclusive* 25, no. 2 (March/April 2006): 61-73.

8. Borger, "Health Spending Projections Through 2015."

9. P. Conrad & V. Leiter, "Medicalisation, Markets and Consumers," *Journal of Health and Social Behavior* 45 (2004): 158-76.

10. P. Starr, *The Social Transformation of American Medicine: The Rise of a Sovereign Profession and the Making of a Vast Industry* (New York: Basic Books, 1984).

11. *The Politics of Cancer* was later expanded and republished in 1998 as *The Politics of Cancer Revisited* by East Ridge Press.

12. *The Cancer Syndrome* was revised in 1996 and published with a new title, *The Cancer Industry,* and was published by Equinox Press.

13. J. Lee, V. Hopkins, & D. Zava. Chapter 1 in *What Your Doctor May Not Tell You About Breast Cancer: How Hormone Balance Can Help Save Your Life* (New York: Warner Books, 2002).

14. D. Davis. *The Secret History of the War on Cancer* (New York: Basic Books, 2007).

15. "Dictionary of Cancer Terms: Cancer," National Cancer Institute. http://www.cancer.gov/dictionary/?CdrID=45333.

16. The Consensus Conference Committee, "Consensus Conference on the Classification of Ductal Carcinoma In Situ," *Cancer* 8, no. 9 (1997): 1798-802; M. J. Silverstein, "Ductal Carcinoma In Situ of the Breast: Controversial Issues," *The Oncologist* 3 (1998): 94-103.

17. H. G. Welch, S. Woloshin, & L. M. Schwartz, "The Sea of Uncertainty Surrounding Ductal Carcinoma In Situ—The Price of Screening Mammography," *Journal of the National Cancer Institute* 100, no. 4 (2008): 228-9.

18. A. Partridge, K. Adloff, E. Blood, et al., "Risk Perceptions and Psychosocial Outcomes of Women with Ductal Carcinoma In Situ: Longitudinal Results from a Cohort Study," *Journal of the National Cancer Institute* 100, no. 4 (2008): 243-51.

19. *Ibid.*

20. Surveillance Epidemiology and End Results, "SEER Fact Sheets: Breast Cancer," National Cancer Institute. http://seer.cancer.gov/statfacts/html/breast.html. All statistics in this report are based on SEER incidence and NCHS mortality statistics. Most can be found within: L. A. G. Ries, D. Melbert, M. Krapcho, et al., eds., *SEER Cancer Statistics Review, 1975–2005,* Bethesda, MD: National Cancer Institute, http://seer.cancer.gov/csr/1975_2005/, based on November 2007 SEER data submission, posted to the SEER Web site, 2008.

21. C. D. Lehman, C. Gatsonis, C. K. Kuhl, et al., "MRI Evaluation of the Contralateral Breast in Women with Recently Diagnosed Breast Cancer," *New England Journal of Medicine* 356, no. 13 (March 2007): 1295-303.

22. S. M. Love, with K. Lindsey, *Dr. Susan Love's Breast Book,* 4th ed. (Cambridge, MA: DaCapo Press), 219.

23. *Ibid.,* 209.

24. *Ibid.,* 209.

25. Partridge, et al., "Risk Perceptions and Psychosocial Outcomes."

26. Love, *Dr. Susan Love's Breast Book,* 209.

27. *Ibid.,* 219; Welch et al., "The Sea of Uncertainty Surrounding Ductal Carcinoma In Situ."

28. "Lobular Carcinoma In Situ (LCIS)," Stanford Medicine. http://cancer.stanford.edu/breastcancer/lcis.html.

29. "Radiation Therapy Helps Prevent DCIS Recurrence After Breast-Conserving Surgery," National Cancer Institute. http://www.cancer.gov/clinicaltrials/results/DCIS0309.

30. "Understanding Breast Cancer Guide: Carcinoma In Situ (LCIS and DCIS)," Susan G. Komen for the Cure. http://ww5.komen.org/BreastCancer/CarcinomainSitu.html.

31. American Cancer Society, *Cancer Facts and Figures 2008.*

32. "Understanding Breast Cancer: Early Detection and Screening," Susan G. Komen for the Cure. http://ww5.komen.org/breastcancer/earlydetectionampscreening.html.

33. J. C. Bailar, "Mammography: A Contrary View," *Annals of Internal Medicine* 84 (1976): 77-84.

34. D. Greenberg, "X-Ray Mammography Background to a Decision," *New England Journal of Medicine* 295, no. 13 (September 23, 1976): 739-40; P. Skrabanek, "False Premises and False Promises of Breast Cancer Screening," *Lancet* 2, no. 8450 (August 10, 1985): 316-20; C. J. Wright & C. B. Mueller, "Screening Mammography and Public Health Policy," *Lancet* 346 (July 1, 1995): 29-32.

35. P. C. Gøtzsche & O. Olsen, "Is Screening for Breast Cancer with Mammography Justifiable?" *Lancet* 355 (January 8, 2000): 129-34. Updated in 2001 in O. Olsen and P. C. Gøtzsche, "Cochrane Review on Screening for Breast Cancer with Mammography," *Lancet* 358, no. 9290 (2001), http://image.thelancet.com/extras/fullreport.pdf; R. Horton, "Screening mammography—an overview revisited," *Lancet* 358, no. 9290 (2001): 1284.

36. Cochrane Database of Systematic Reviews 2006, s.v. "Screening for Breast Cancer with Mammography" (P. C. Gøtzsche and M. Nielsen), http://www.cochrane.org/reviews/en/ab001877.html.

37. L. L. Humphrey, M. Helfand, B. K. Chan, et al., "Breast Cancer Screening: A Summary of the Evidence for the U.S. Preventive Services Task Force," *Annals of Internal Medicine* 137 (2002): 347-60.

38. K. Armstrong, E. Moye, S. Williams, et al., "Screening Mammography in Women 40 to 49 Years of Age: A Systematic Review

for the American College of Physicians," *Annals of Internal Medicine* 146, no. 7 (April 13, 2007): 516-26.

39. Institute of Medicine, *Mammography and Beyond: Developing Technologies for the Early Detection of Breast Cancer* (Washington, DC: National Academy Press, 2001), 13.

40. A. von Eschenbach., Testimony to the U. S. Senate Committee on Appropriations Subcommittee on Labor, Health and Human Services, Education, and Related Agencies and the Committee on Health, Education, Labor and Pensions Subcommittee on Public Health, on February 28, 2002. National Cancer Institute. http://legislative.cancer.gov/hearings/research#2002.

41. D. A. Berry, K. A. Cronin, S. K. Plevritis, et al., for the Cancer Intervention and Surveillance Modeling Network (CISNET) Collaborators, "Effect of Screening and Adjuvant Therapy on Mortality from Breast Cancer," *New England Journal of Medicine* 353 (2005): 1784-92. http://www.cancer.gov/newscenter/pressreleases/CISNET#1; G. Kolata. "Mammograms Validated as Key In Cancer Fight," *New York Times*, October 27, 2005.

42. "Clinical Trials: Get the Facts About Cancer Screening Studies," National Cancer Institute. http://cancerweb.ncl.ac.uk/cancernet/600530.html.

43. L. Nyström, I. Andersson, N. Bjurstam, et al., "Long-Term Effects of Mammography Screening: Updated Overview of the Swedish Randomised Trials," *Lancet* 359 (2002): 909-19; A. Barratt, K. Howard, L. Irwig, et al., "Model of Outcomes of Screening Mammography: Information to Support Informed Choices," *British Medical Journal* 330, no. 7497 (2005): 936-8; L. M. Schwartz & S. Woloshin, "Participation in Mammography Screening," *British Medical Journal* 335, no. 7623 (2007): 731; Cochrane Database, Gøtzsche & Nielsen, "Screening for Breast Cancer with Mammography."

44. A. Qaseem, V. Snow, K. Sherif, et al., "Screening Mammography for Women 40–49 Years of Age: A Clinical Practice Guideline from the American College of Physicians," *Annals of Internal Medicine* 146 (2007): 511-5.

45. P. C. Gøtzsche, O. J. Hartling, M. Nielsen, et al., "Breast Screening: The Facts—Or Maybe Not," *British Medical Journal* 338, no. b86 (2009): 338-448.

46. U.S. Preventative Task Force. "Screening for Breast Cancer: U.S. Preventive Services Task Force Recommendation Statement." *Annals of Internal Medicine* 151 (2009): 1-44.

47. "Detailed Guide: Breast Cancer—Can Breast Cancer Be Found Early?" American Cancer Society. http://www.cancer.org/docroot/CRI/content/CRI_2_4_3X_Can_breast_cancer_be_found_early_5.asp.

48. "American Cancer Society Responds to Changes to USPSTF Mammography Guidelines." American Cancer Society. http://www.cancer.org/docroot/MED/content/MED_2_1x_American_Cancer_Society_Responds_to_Changes_to_USPSTF_Mammography_Guidelines.asp

49. H. L. Howe, P. A. Wingo, M. J. Thun, et al., "Annual Report to the Nation on the Status of Cancer (1973 through 1998), Featuring Cancers with Recent Increasing Trends," *Journal of the National Cancer Institute* 93, no. 11 (2001): 824-42.

50. L. A. G. Ries, M. P. Eisner, C. L. Kosary, et al., eds., *SEER Fast Stats: Breast Cancer 1994–2003*, (Bethesda, MD: National Cancer Institute, 2006).

51. Institute of Medicine, "Mammography and Beyond," Washington, DC: National Academy Press, 2001, 39.

52. C. Christensen, F. Wang, M. B. Barton, et al., "Predicting the Cumulative Risk of False-positive Mammograms," *Journal of the National Cancer Institute* 92, no. 20 (2000): 1657-66.

53. "Relative Cost of Different Breast Biopsy Methods," Imaginis: The Women's Health Resource. http://www.imaginis.com/breast-health/biopsy/general2.asp.

54. Office on Women's Health. U.S. Department of Health and Human Services, "Health Insurance and Women," womenshealth.gov. http://www.4women.gov/faq/health-insurance-women.cfm.

55. J. A. Harvey, L. L. Fajardo, & C. A. Innis, "Previous Mammograms in Patients with Impalpable Breast Carcinoma: Retrospective vs. Blinded Interpretation," *AJR American Journal of Roentgenology*, 161 (1993): 1167-72; J. A. Van Digck, A. L. Verbeek, L. Beex, et al., "The Current Detectability of Breast Cancer in a Mammographic Screening Program. A Review of the Previous Mammograms of Interval and Screen-Detectd Cancers. *Cancer*, 72 (1993): 1933-8; L. J. Warren Burhenne, S. A. Wood, C. J. D'Orsi, et al, "Potential Contribution of Computer-Aided Detection to the Sensitivity of Screening Mammography," *Radiology* 216, no. 1 (2000): 54-62; I. Saarenmaa et al., "The Visibility of Cancer on Previous Mammograms in Retrospective Review," *Clinical Radiology* 56, no. 1 (2001): 40-3.

56. J. J. James, A. J. Evans, S. E. Pinder, et al., "Is the Presence of Mammographic Comedo Calcification Really a Prognostic Factor for Small Screen-Detected Invasive Breast Cancers?" *Clinical Radiology* 58, no. 1 (2003): 54-62.

57. D. L. Miglioretti, R. Smith-Bindman, L. Abraham, et al., "Radiologist Characteristics Associated With Interpretive Performance of Diagnostic Mammography," *Journal of the National Cancer Institute*, 99 (2007): 1854-63.

58. Love, *Dr. Susan Love's Breast Book.*

59. .V. L. Ernster, J. Barclay, K. Kerlikowske, D. Grady, & I. C. Henderson, "Incidence of and Treatment for Ductal Carcinoma In Situ of the Breast," *Journal of the American Medical Association*, 275 (1996), no. 12: 913-8.

60. Cochrane Database, Gøtzsche & Nielsen, "Screening for Breast Cancer with Mammography."

61. J. Lee, D. Zava, & V. Hopkins, "Per-Henrik Zahl and Jan Mæhlen Model of Outcomes of Screening Mammography: Spontaneous Regression of Breast Cancer May Not Be Uncommon," *British Medical Journal* 331, no. 7512 (2005): 350; Lee, Hopkins, & Zava, *What Your Doctor May Not Tell You About Breast Cancer.*

62. Welch, Woloshin, & Schwartz, "The Sea of Uncertainty Surrounding Ductal Carcinoma"; J. Huang & W. J. Mackillop, "Increased Risk of Soft Tissue Sarcoma After Radiotherapy in Women with Breast Carcinoma," *Cancer* 92 (2001): 532-6; J. Gray, ed., "State of the Evidence 2008: The Connection Between Breast Cancer and the Environment," Breast Cancer Fund and Breast Cancer Action. (San Francisco, CA: Cooperative Printing, 2008); J. W. Gofman, *Preventing Breast Cancer: The Story of a Major, Proven, Preventable Cause of This Disease,* 2nd ed. (San Francisco: Committee for Nuclear Responsibility Book Division, 1996); J. W. Gofman, *Radiation from Medical Procedures in the Pathogenesis of Cancer and Ischemic Heart Disease: Dose-Response Studies with Physicians per 100,000 Population* (San Francisco: Committee for Nuclear Responsibility Book Division, 1999).

63. P. H. Zahl, B. H. Strand, & J. Mæhlen, "Incidence of Breast Cancer in Norway and Sweden During Introduction of Nationwide Screening: Prospective Cohort Study," *British Medical Journal* 328 (2004): 921-4.

64. Food and Drug Administration, "Reducing Radiation from Medical X-rays." U. S. Department of Health and Human Services. http://www.fda.gov/ForConsumers/ConsumerUpdates/ucm095505.htm.

65. S. Epstein, R. Bertell, & B. Seaman, et al., "Dangers and Unreliability of Mammography: Breast Examination Is a Safe, Effective, and Practical Alternative," *International Journal of Health Services* 31, no. 3 (2001): 605-15.

66. A. Berrington de Gonzalez, C. D. Berg, K. Visvanathan, et al., "Estimated Risk of Radiation-Induced Breast Cancer from Mammographic Screening for Young BRCA Mutation Carriers," *Journal of the National Cancer Institute* 101, no. 3 (2009): 205-9; B. Friedenson, "Is Mammography Indicated for Women With Defective BRCA Genes? Implications of Recent Scientific Advances for the Diagnosis, Treatment, and Prevention of Hereditary Breast Cancer," *Medscape General Medicine* 2, no. 1 (2000): E9. http://www.ncbi.nlm.nih.gov/pubmed/11104455.

67. K. J. Jorgensen & P. C. Gøtzsche, "Content of Invitations to Publicly Funded Screening Mammography," *British Medical Journal* 332 (2006): 538-41.

68. Gøtzsche et al., "Breast Screening"

69. Gøtzsche et al., "Breast Screening"

70. "Find a Komen Affiliate," Susan G. Komen for the Cure. http://ww5.komen.org/affiliates.aspx.

71. "Accuracy of Mammograms," Susan G. Komen for the Cure. http://ww5.komen.org/BreastCancer/AccuracyofMammograms.html.

72. G. A. Sulik, "Managing Biomedical Uncertainty: The Techno-scientific Illness Identity," *Sociology of Health and Illness* 31, no. 7 (2009): 1-18.

73. N. Breen, K. A. Cronin, H. I. Meissner, et al., "Reported Drop in Mammography: Is This Cause for Concern?" *Cancer* 109, no. 12 (2007): 2405-9.

74. "Fact Sheet. Screening Mammograms: Questions and Answers," National Cancer Institute. http://www.cancer.gov/cancertopics/factsheet/detection/screening-mammograms.

75. "Mammogram," National Women's Law Center. http://hrc.nwlc.org/Policy-Indicators/Addressing-Wellness-and-Prevention/Mammogram.aspx. The *Report Card* uses annual screenings for women age 40 and older as its standard to determine whether states meet the policy because it is the age at which the American Cancer Society recommends

women begin annual mammograms. "Cancer Detection Guidelines," American Cancer Society. http://www.cancer.org/docroot/ped/content/ped_2_3x_acs_cancer_detection_guidelines_36.asp.

76. U. S. Census Bureau, Census 2000: Detailed Tables. http://factfinder.census.gov/servlet/DTTable?_bm=y&-geo_id=01000US&-ds_name=DEC_2000_SF1_U&-_lang=en&-mt_name=DEC_2000_SF1_U_P012&-format=&-CONTEXT=dt.

77. Department of Health and Human Services, National Breast and Cervical Cancer Early Detection Program, Centers for Disease Control and Prevention. http://apps.nccd.cdc.gov/cancercontacts/nbccedp/contactlist.asp.

78. U.S. Department of Health and Human Services, "National Breast and Cervical Cancer Early Detection Program: 1991–2002 National Report," Centers for Disease Control and Prevention. http://www.cdc.gov/cancer/nbccedp/Reports/NationalReport/index.htm.

79. "Cost Analysis of the National Breast and Cervical Cancer Early Detection Program: Selected States, 2003 to 2004," *Cancer* 112 (2008): 626-35. http://www.ncbi.nlm.nih.gov/pubmed/18157831.

80. J. Whitney, "A Clear Picture: Top Imaging Companies Share Their Perspectives on Industry Advancements and What's to Come," *Medical Product Outsourcing Magazine*, April 1, 2007. http://www.mpo-mag.com/articles/2007/04/a-clear-picture.

81. Digital Mammographic Imaging Screening Trial (DMIST) Investigators Group, "Diagnostic Performance of Digital versus Film Mammography for Breast-Cancer Screening," *New England Journal of Medicine* 353, no. 17 (2005): 1773-83.

82. "GE Healthcare's Innovation and Multi-Modality Technologies Advancing Breast Cancer Care," GE Healthcare. http://www.gehealthcare.com/company/pressroom/releases/pr_release_10365.html.

83. *Ibid.*

84. "Initiatives," Breast Cancer Help, Inc., http://www.breastcancer-helpinc.org/initiatives.php.

85. D. Lidor, "Infoimaging: Digital Mammography Better Than X-Rays," *Forbes*, September 16, 2005. http://www.forbes.com/2005/09/16/digital-mammography-screening-cx_dl_0916digital.html.

86. IMS HEALTH Incorporated, Top-line Industry Data, 2008 Global Prescription Sales Information, "Global Pharmaceutical Sales, 2001-2008," IMS National Sales Perspectives. http://www.imshealth.com/portal/site/imshealth/menuitem.a46c6d4df3db4b3d88f611019418c22a/?vgnextoid=cec0977ccedc0210VgnVCM100000ed152ca2RCRD&cpsext currchannel=1

87. The Henry J. Kaiser Family Foundation, *Prescription Drug Trends Fact Sheet:* Publication Number 3057-07 (Healthcare Marketplace Project, November 9, 2008).

88. *Ibid.*

89. "Pharmacy Benefit Management: PBM Market Share," AIS Market Data. http://www.aishealth.com/MarketData/PharmBenMgmt/PBM_market02.html.

90. IMS, "IMS Health Forecasts Continued Double-Digit Annual Growth of Cancer Therapeutics: Global Sales Expected to Exceed $75 Billion by 2012," news release, May 15, 2008.

91. "Pfizer Reviews Progress of Oncology Pipeline and New Commercial Business Unit Structure with Analysts," *Business Wire*, June 2, 2008. http://findarticles.com/p/articles/mi_m0EIN/is_2008_June_2/ai_n25472806/

92. "2008 Annual Report," GlaxoSmithKline. http://www.gsk.com/reportsandpublications.htm.

93. *Ibid.;* "GSK shakes up R&D," *Fierce Biotech Newsletter*, December 12, 2007. http://www.fiercebiotech.com/story/gsk-shakes-r-d/2007-12-12.

94. "AstraZeneca Receives Six Months Pediatric Exclusivity Patent Extension for ARIMIDEX(R)(anastrozole) from the FDA," bio-medicine. org. http://www.bio-medicine.org/medicine-news-1/AstraZeneca-Receives-Six-Months-Pediatric-Exclusivity-Patent-Extension-for-ARIMIDEX-28R-29—28anastrozole-29-from-the-FDA-7263-1/.

95. Media Education Foundation. *Big Bucks, Big Pharma: Marketing Disease and Pushing Drugs*. 60 Masonic St., Northampton, MA 01060 (a documentary).

96. Center for Drug Evaluation and Research, "Electronic Orange Book: Approved Drug Products with Therapeutic Equivalence Evaluations," Food and Drug Administration. www.fda.gov/cder/ob/.

97. T. Fojo & C. Grady, "How Much Is Life Worth: Cetuximab, Non–Small Cell Lung Cancer, and the $440 Billion Question," *Journal of the National Cancer Institute* 101 (2009): 1-5.

98. C. Arnst, "Soaring Cancer Drug Costs May Cripple Medicare," *Business Week*, January 27, 2009, www.businessweek.com.

99. P. Bach, "Limits on Medicare's Ability to Control Rising Spending on Cancer Drugs," *New England Journal of Medicine* 360, no. 6 (February 5): 626-33.

100. W. P. Peters, G. Rosner, & J. Vredenburgh, "A Prospective, Randomized Comparison of Two Doses of Combination Alkyating Agents (AA) as Consolidation after CAF in High-Risk Primary Breast Cancer Involving Ten or More Axillary Lymph Nodes (LN): Preliminary Results of CALGB 9082/SWOG 9114/NCIC MA-13," (paper presented at the American Society of Clinical Oncology Annual Meeting, San Francisco, CA, May 12-15, 1999).

101. W. R. Bezwoda, "Randomised, Controlled Trial of High Dose Chemotherapy (HD-CNVp) versus Standard Dose (CAF) Chemotherapy for High Risk, Surgically Treated, Primary Breast Cancer," (paper presented

at the American Society of Clinical Oncology Annual Meeting, San Francisco, CA, May 12-15, 1999).

102. E. A. Stadtmauer, A. O'Neill, & L. J. Goldstein, "Conventional-Dose Chemotherapy Compared with High-Dose Chemotherapy Plus Autologous Hematopoietic Stem-Cell Transplantation for Metastatic Breast Cancer," *New England Journal of Medicine* 342, no. 15 (2000): 1069-76; J. P. Lotz, H. Cure, & M. Janvier, "High-Dose Chemotherapy (HD-CT) with Hematopoietic Stem Cells Transplantation (HSCT) for Metastatic Breast Cancer (MBC): Results of the French Protocol PEGASE 04" (paper presented at the American Society of Clinical Oncology Annual Meeting, Atlanta, GA, May 15-18, 1999).

103. L. Johnson, "Hormone Therapy Sales Off 52 Percent," *Associated Press,* November 14, 2002. http://health.groups.yahoo.com/group/iatrogenic/message/782.

104. G. A. Colditz, S. E. Hankinson, & D. J. Hunter, "The Use of Estrogens and Progestins and the Risk of Breast Cancer in Postmenopausal Women," *New England Journal of Medicine* 332 (1995): 1589-93.

105. The Writing Group for the PEPI Trial, "Effects of Estrogen or Estrogen/Progestin Regimens on Heart Disease Risk Factors in Postmenopausal Women: The Post Menopausal Estrogen/Progestin Interventions Trial," *Journal of the American Medical Association,* 273 (1995): 199-208.

106. M. Stone, "Hormone-Replacement Therapy and Breast Cancer," *CNN.com,* May 26, 1999. http://www.cnn.com/HEALTH/cancer/9905/26/hrt.breast.cancer/.

107. Writing Group for the Women's Health Initiative Investigators, "Risks and Benefits of Estrogen Plus Progestin in Healthy Postmenopausal Women: Principal Results From the Women's Health Initiative Randomized Controlled Trial," *Journal of the American Medical Association* 288 (2002): 321-33. Until recently, the only data supporting HRT's use came

from observational studies of voluntary behavior—studies that compared women who chose to take HRT with women who chose not to. These studies found that the women who took HRT had fewer heart attacks and strokes and were less likely to develop osteoporosis. Because these studies were observational in nature, they could not answer the question of whether HRT made women healthy or whether healthy women took HRT. To determine whether HRT was effective, in 1993 the National Institutes of Health began the WHI, the first long-term, randomized, placebo-controlled study designed to measure the benefits and risks of HRT use. Randomized placebo-controlled trials are the gold standard of medical research because, unlike observational studies, they can prove cause and effect. More than 16,000 women between the ages of 50 and 79 were enrolled between 1993 and 1998 in the WHI trial. Half of the women were given HRT; the other half were given a placebo.

108. Johnson, "Hormone Therapy Sales Off 52 Percent."

109. According to ACS "Breast Cancer Facts & Figures 2005–2006" and the "Status of Cancer" report co-released by the National Cancer Institute (NCI), American Cancer Society (ACS), Centers for Disease Control (CDC), and the North American Association of Central Cancer Registries (NAACCR); P. Radvin et al., "The Decrease in Breast-Cancer Incidence in 2003 in the United States," *New England Journal of Medicine*, 356 (2007): 1670-74.

110. Johnson, "Hormone Therapy Sales Off 52 Percent."

111. M. Bellisle, "Former Wyeth Pharmaceutical Rep Testifies Company Downplayed Risks," *Reno Gazette-Journal*, September 13, 2007, A3.

112. Fred Hutchinson Cancer Research Center, "Combined Hormone Replacement Therapy Increases Risk Of Lobular Breast Cancer Fourfold After Just 3 Years Of Use," *Science Daily,* January 16, 2008. http://www.sciencedaily.com/releases/2008/01/080115085403.htm (accessed December 9, 2008).

113. K. Niland, "Wyeth Developing Another HRT for Menopause," Beasley, Allen, Crow, Methvin, Portis & Miles, P.C. http://www.hrt-legal.com/news/2008/10/02/wyeth-developing-another-hrt-for-menopause/.

114. M. Klawiter, "Racing for the Cure, Walking Women, and Toxic Touring," in *Health and Health Care as Social Problems,* eds. P. Conrad & V. Leiter, 161-88 (Lanham, MD: Rowman and Littlefield, 2003), 175.

115. "About NBCAM." National Breast Cancer Awareness Month. http://nbcam.org/about_nbcam.cfm. NBCAM reports 2,375,058 visitors between January 1, 2007, and February 12, 2009.

116. "Sample Press Release," National Breast Cancer Awareness Month. http://nbcam.org/help_downloads.cfm.

117. "New GE Cordless Phone Raises Funds for National Breast Cancer Foundation," GE Communications Solutions. http://www.home-electronics.net/ge/pc/viewContent.asp?idpage=14.

118. M. Napoli, "GE's Misleading Ad Campaign for Digital Mammography," Healthfacts. Center for Medical Consumers, Inc. http://findarticles.com/p/articles/mi_mo815/is_2001_Oct/ai_78900349/.

119. P. Conrad, *The Medicalization of Society: On the Transformation of Human Conditions to Treatable Disorders* (Baltimore, MD: The Johns Hopkins University Press, 2007).

120. AstraZeneca advertisement in *Ladies' Home Journal,* October 2002, 99.

121. King, *Pink Ribbons, Inc.,* 81–82.

122. Brystol-Meyers Squibb, Facility Information, Lawrenceville, New Jersey. "Civic activities supported," http://www.ifex.com/static/ehs/facili/data/lawren.html

123. "International Conference Convenes Young Breast Cancer Survivors, Leading Healthcare Experts to Address Breast Cancer in Young Women," Susan G. Komen for the Cure. http://ww5.komen.org/KomenNewsArticle.aspx?id=7460.

SIX

UNDER THE PINK
Optimism, Selfishness, and Guilt

Emotional labor...requires one to induce or suppress feeling in order to sustain the outward countenance that produces the proper state of mind in others.
ARLIE HOCHSCHILD, THE MANAGED HEART[1]

RUBY'S STORY

Three weeks before her 46th birthday, Ruby went for a routine mammogram. The slides suggested suspicious calcifications. Breast calcifications are common as women age, and most of the time (98 percent) they reflect a benign process. Sometimes calcifications are categorized as "indeterminate" or "suspicious." Though these types of calcifications also tend to be benign, they are sometimes an early sign of breast cancer. It is common for radiologists to request a second mammogram to confirm the classification, and this was what happened in Ruby's case. As an oncology nurse, she knew that this process was routine and rationally concluded that it was nothing to worry about. Still, there was a degree of uncertainty that was troubling. Ruby told no one of her concern and scheduled the second mammogram. In the meantime, she went on with her daily routine, attended a family wedding, and tried not to think about it.

On the day of her 46th birthday, Ruby had the second mammogram. Comparing her mammograms from the previous 3 years, the doctor explained that the group of "suspicious" cells had become larger and darker over time. He believed that this change on the X-ray slides represented either a tumor that started to grow 3 years earlier, or an area of dense tissue that was getting denser as Ruby aged. The doctor gave Ruby the option of waiting for 6 months and having another mammogram, or having a biopsy to establish whether the tissue in that area was benign. Ruby did not want to wait, so the doctor wrote the order for a biopsy. The decision to have a breast biopsy rather than taking a "wait and watch" approach is related to the sense of fear and urgency surrounding the early detection of breast cancer. However, waiting for biopsy results affects stress hormone levels (i.e., cortisol) just as much as finding out you have breast cancer.[2] Ruby's anxiety mounted.

By the time Ruby got home, she was not thinking about the birthday dinner she had planned with her family. She was anxious to tell her partner and her adult children about the biopsy and was nervous about how they would respond. As Ruby talked about dinner plans and waited for her son's arrival, she was preoccupied with the impending announcement. She wanted to tell her children at the same time, but when she looked around the room to see her partner and her daughter, she blurted out: "Both of you are here, so I might as well tell you something! I want you to sit down and not worry about it, but I just had a second mammogram today and [have a] biopsy scheduled [for] ten days from now." Ruby's daughter asked how long this had been going on, and Ruby replied, "Not long. I just found out today." Ruby's answer was perplexing: if this were her *second* mammogram, then she must have had a *first* mammogram. When was the first one? Why did Ruby keep it to herself? Ruby's daughter pressed for information, and Ruby explained that she had the first mammogram prior to the wedding. She said, "It was inconclusive… That's why I went for a second one. I did not tell anybody because of the wedding. And, there was nothing to say."

Some personal feelings happen in the gut, as people respond on an emotional level to physical experiences, events, interactions with others, and the content of one's imagination. There are few words to express the emotions of the subtle body. Other feelings are conscientiously evaluated, organized, and used to manage social relationships and construct a coherent sense of self. This chapter, which is concerned with the latter, considers how the emotions of diagnosed women are embedded within social expectations about *how to feel*. In Ruby's case, she did not want talk of mammograms to interfere with a wedding celebration. Still, the wedding had come and gone, and she still told no one about it because *there was nothing to say*. This phrase suggests that there were no words to express what Ruby felt. In addition to the gut-wrenching shock associated with life-threatening illness,

Ruby's emotions were related to her social roles—as an oncology nurse, as a mother of two adult children, as a 46-year-old divorced woman, and as a woman who may be facing breast cancer. These roles intersected with expectations about gender, age, medicine, and cancer culture. As Ruby and other diagnosed women make sense of breast cancer, social context supplies the rules of engagement.

Arlie Hochschild explains that conventions of feeling, or feeling rules, govern what people think and do, about how they feel (i.e., the *"shoulds"* and *"should nots"* about how to feel in particular situations, such as being happy at weddings and crying at funerals). Feeling rules provide a benchmark for gauging how to feel about social roles, relationships, bodies, and illnesses. Although people routinely negotiate, transgress, and sometimes alter social norms, societies have ways of encouraging and enforcing what they view as appropriate. Social context shapes public understandings of breast cancer, establishes the rules of survivorship, and promotes a specific framework for dealing with the illness that includes conventions of feeling.

The first part of this book mapped the social context of breast cancer. Chapter 2 examined the role of the breast cancer movement in shaping the development of a pink ribbon culture. Chapter 3 analyzed the competing masculine and feminine ethos within the broader U.S. cancer culture, which provides gendered role models and principles of survivorship. Pink ribbon culture constructs an idealized model of survivorship (embodied in the image of the "she-ro"), which integrates these seemingly opposed gender mores. The proliferation of breast cancer in mass media and public culture, discussed in Chapter 4, disseminates information and cultural knowledge as images and narratives that encourage open disclosure, commitment to the cause, pink consumption, solidarity, and the valorization of the she-ro. Chapter 5 considered the role of medical consumerism in maintaining pink ribbon culture and the breast cancer industry as a distinct medical market. To understand breast cancer, we must understand the role of social context in shaping the ideological and emotional work involved in women's responses to it.

"BECOMING" A BREAST CANCER SURVIVOR: LEARNING THE RULES

Michael Bury argues that chronic illness disrupts not only a person's everyday life but also the explanatory systems that sustain it. Individuals develop coping strategies to manage disruption, evaluate taken-for-granted assumptions and behaviors, and reconsider their self-concept and personal biography.[3] *Becoming a breast cancer survivor* thereby involves the development of an illness identity and the (re)writing of one's personal biography—one that takes the illness, social expectations, and feeling rules into account. The "shoulds" and "should nots" of survivorship are visible within the personal biography, illuminating the social and cultural factors that underlie women's responses to breast cancer. A variety of social expectations, interpersonal relations,

and cultural representations enhance and/or constrain the feeling rules, revealing the serious emotional work[4] involved in
maintaining them.

In this chapter, I present the feeling rules of breast cancer
survivorship as an overarching framework to analyze the impact
of social context on women's experiences of breast cancer and
sense of self. The feeling rules often occur simultaneously, and
encourage specific behaviors, coping mechanisms, and cultural
repertoires.

- Feeling Rule 1: Survivorship requires a strong sense of *optimism* in terms of hope, faith, and transcendence.
- Feeling Rule 2: Survivorship necessitates *selfishness,* which is
  constructed in masculine terms as a rational coping strategy or as a confession of gender violations related to wom-
  en's nurturance and selflessness.
- Feeling Rule 3: *Guilt* results from the stigma associated
  with failing to present oneself adequately as a she-roic survivor, losing bodily integrity, or disrupting gender roles.

Ruby's early diagnosis experience sets the stage for exploring
how women develop an illness identity in relation to the feeling
rules of survivorship. The accounts profiled in this chapter, and
in the next one, are drawn from a sample of 60 breast cancer
survivors, aged 31 to 79 years, who were interviewed from 2001
to 2003. The years of survivorship range from 1 year (22 percent)
to 10 or more years (13 percent), with the greatest percentage of
women in the 2- to 4-year range (42 percent). Their narratives

demonstrate common themes among breast cancer survivors as they develop their personal breast cancer biography.

FEELING RULE 1: OPTIMISM

Feeling rules necessitate responses to illness through a dichotomous system of appraisal that provides a benchmark for evaluating behavior. The primary feeling rule for achieving she-ro status in pink ribbon culture is optimism. Cultural representations construct optimism through displays of hope, faith, and transcendence. She-roes successfully display optimism by normalizing their experiences, avoiding complaints, and using breast cancer as a catalyst for empowerment. The expectation for unequivocal cheerfulness requires emotional restraint. Pink ribbon culture, and much of Western culture, values such self-control, but it takes considerable emotional work to conceal feelings of anxiety, depression, concern, or pain. Women's responses to this feeling rule represent two ends of the optimism spectrum.

Incorporation of the She-ro

Personal narratives illustrate a progression of feelings and accompanying actions that ultimately result in the incorporation of key aspects of the she-ro model. Roslyn's story parallels many women's accounts. The elements of Roslyn's story that center on optimism are most likely to be the aspects of her experience that would be featured in survivor profiles, news articles, and other cultural representations of breast cancer in pink ribbon culture. Here is a synopsis.

Roslyn separated from her husband 6 months before she was diagnosed with breast cancer. Although she had assumed for many years that she was responsible for her husband's alcoholism, Roslyn eventually decided that she no longer wanted to be married. She believed that she had an obligation to stay in the marriage until she had fulfilled her responsibilities, which centered on raising her children in a two-parent home until they reached adulthood. When Roslyn's son was 30 and her daughter was in her twenties, Roslyn was ready to leave her husband and start a new life. Then, she "got hit with [breast cancer]." Roslyn had a tendency to feel responsible for things that were outside of her control, such as her husband's drinking. Likewise, her immediate response to a breast cancer diagnosis was to feel like it was her fault. She said, "I got cancer...because I left [my husband] when I shouldn't have...what did I do?" Roslyn thought her diagnosis was punishment for ending her marriage.

Roslyn's breast cancer diagnosis brought gender relations to the surface. After being married for 30 years, she was practiced in putting the needs of others first. She was afraid of being alone, unsure of her decisions, and felt unsettled at the prospect of depending upon those she had once nurtured, especially her children. She even considered returning to the marriage she had just ended. She said, "I almost went back to my husband because

I thought, 'I can't do this by myself…and I don't want to depend on my kids…they've got their own lives…'" A commitment to traditional gender roles can make it difficult for women to face breast cancer on their own terms even as breast cancer can disrupt the nurturing roles that women value.

As an added stressor, many people initially believe that breast cancer is a death sentence. Roslyn was diagnosed in October, but she was convinced that she would not survive the year. She packed her summer clothes to donate to Goodwill and called her employer's human resources department to cancel her retirement. Roslyn had seen the mortality statistics, and she personally knew of people who had died. She felt alone, overwhelmed, and fatalistic. The human resources manager asked Roslyn to take a few days to reconsider before canceling her retirement. Roslyn heeded this advice and came to the realization that she could not anticipate what her treatment would entail or how long she would live. She unpacked her summer clothes and refrained from canceling her retirement.

During the early phase of a cancer diagnosis, fear and uncertainty are paramount. The desire to normalize one's experience is a common coping mechanism for people with varied diseases and chronic conditions. For breast cancer, optimism is a key facet of normalization that stresses self-presentation and composure. In social interaction, breast cancer should not interfere with one's life or anyone else's. Likewise, Roslyn was fearful but had internalized these aspects of the survivor model early on. She maintained normalcy by keeping her diagnosis and her concerns to herself, something she framed as self-reliance. This is how she explained it:

> I was not dealing well with my diagnosis. I think one of the reasons…was because I… really didn't want anyone to know. I thought, it's my problem, not their problem…If I just don't talk about it…everything will be fine. Well, it wasn't fine… I needed to vent.

After 2 years of keeping her diagnosis quiet, Roslyn eventually did what most people do: she incorporated breast cancer into her life and her sense of self.

Pink ribbon culture confers status on those who publicly claim triumphant survivorship. As women interact regularly with other survivors, it often becomes easier to identify with the culture's version of survivorship. Women who share their story openly, attend support groups, and think of themselves as "survivors" are more likely to view breast cancer as a catalyst for empowerment, and she-roic survivorship as a valued illness identity. Roslyn is now known at work as the "go-to" person for information about breast cancer. She attends support groups regularly, participates in breast cancer awareness campaigns, runs in the Komen race every year, and is proud to wear pink. Self-reflective empathy is one of the reasons Roslyn does these things. She said, "It's important for women to know that I'm here, and I'm talking about it…I have a list of people I call every week… I didn't have anyone to call [me] and say, 'you're gonna be okay.'" She-roic survivorship offers women like Roslyn a new nurturing role that is altruistic and reinforcing of their illness identity.

When women start to think of breast cancer as a catalyst for empowerment, it opens the possibility for building a new sense of individuation and self-realization as women. Choosing to exhibit pink femininity with pride confers social value to traditionally feminine attributes while recontextualizing them in terms of survivorship. The breast cancer experience frequently demarcates a transitional point in women's perceptions of themselves. Roslyn is no exception. In her account, she describes herself *before* breast cancer as innately weak, agreeable, compliant, and fearful. *After* breast cancer, she describes herself in she-roic terms—with strength, determination, assertiveness, courage, and pride.

> Never in my wildest dreams did I think I could be a strong person, because I'm not a strong person…I never was. I was just, "okay, okay, okay"…I would do anything to avoid an argument. I don't like confrontation. But, I stand up for my health now.

When Roslyn interjects the present tense in the midst of describing herself in the past ("Because I'm not a strong person…I never was"), it suggests that she still feels weak to a degree. Taking proactive and responsible action on behalf of her health is a vital aspect of developing the valued characteristics of the she-ro, which seeped into other aspects of her life. Roslyn went on to say, "I'm very confident at work now…even got a new job…should have done it 20 years ago." Roslyn has the spirit and optimism that embodies she-roic survivorship.

People feel good about making changes in their lives that they, and others, view as positive. Critical medical diagnoses and other life-changing events give individuals a reason to change aspects of their lives that they may have wanted to change for a long time. Roslyn is pleased with what she has done, and who she has become, in response to breast cancer. She went from hiding her diagnosis to sharing it openly. She countered fear with solidarity, hope, and transcendence. She readily shares her story with other women and has ongoing relationships with other survivors. The highlights of Roslyn's story could be molded easily to the she-roic tale—a dramatic cancer story that ultimately ends with the she-ro being a better person and having a better life. In doing so, this popular story leaves out key aspects to women's experiences.

In my conversations with breast cancer survivors, women frequently captured the optimism embedded within their stories in the word "blessing." If we had stopped the conversation there, I might have thought they were referring to a miracle or stroke of good fortune. This was not what most women meant. Instead, the blessing was about permission: breast cancer permitted women to take on a new and valued identity. I asked Roslyn if she counted breast cancer as a blessing and she replied:

> I would never call [breast cancer] a blessing…but, it brought me through different stages in my life…and maybe I wouldn't be as strong as I am today had this not happened to me… I needed to get some strength. I didn't want to, particularly, get it this way.

The upbeat message of breast cancer survivorship provides a counterbalance to the feelings of fear and uncertainty that accompany diagnosis and treatment. The simplistic overemphasis on normalization, transcendence, and empowerment in pink ribbon culture obscures this complexity. The mandate for optimism involves an aesthetic approach to normalization through appearance and self-presentation, which integrates social expectations for women's conciliatory behavior, specifically the suppression of any feelings that might destabilize upbeat social interaction. Many diagnosed women refuse to participate in pink ribbon culture precisely for this reason.

Rejecting the She-ro

Fifty-seven-year-old Barbara was among the first women I formally interviewed for this research. Her story, though common, garners little representation in mass media or pink ribbon culture. If Roslyn's narrative represents the high end of the optimism spectrum, Barbara's would represent the low end. Many women on this end of the continuum discuss social and cultural barriers to defining and expressing survivorship in ways that are meaningful to them. This theme was striking in my conversation with Barbara, whose experience was more vivid because of her background. Barbara's twin sister was diagnosed with breast cancer (a known risk factor for ovarian cancer) and died from ovarian cancer at age 45. After Barbara's sister was diagnosed with these cancers, many people urged Barbara to have a prophylactic procedure to reduce her risk. Medical consumerism encourages proactive and responsible behavior to prevent disease and restore health, which sometimes involves making decisions about removing a healthy part of the body for preventive reasons. For many women, the removal of a reproductive body part (such as the breast, uterus, or ovaries) involves considerations about whether they have, or want to have, biological children. Although apprehensive, Barbara agreed to have a hysterectomy because she already had two children and was beyond her childbearing years.

Knowing that Barbara's sister had been diagnosed with breast cancer prior to ovarian cancer, Barbara's doctor suggested that she also have a prophylactic mastectomy. According to Barbara, he said: "While you're at it, have your breasts scooped out." During the interview, I was troubled by the imagery and word choice, thinking to myself that the doctor's suggestion seemed inappropriate and unsympathetic. Since Barbara was recounting her conversation from memory, the word "scooped" may have been Barbara's word and not her doctor's. Regardless, it was clear that the doctor was recommending proactive action in the form of a prophylactic procedure, and that his recommendation had a major impact on Barbara's perspective. Barbara said, "I couldn't do it then. I was newly divorced. They had reconstruction... I would have been a good candidate. But, I didn't really think about it."

Barbara's statement reveals a cultural facet to her decision that goes beyond biology and reproduction. In Western society, women's breasts symbolize femininity and female sexuality. Damage to, or removal of, the breasts is aberrant in a heteronormative culture that is "obsessed with breasts."[5] For this reason, women may prefer breast-conserving surgeries, especially if they are younger, childless, or single. Although reproduction was no longer a concern for Barbara, she was newly divorced and felt pressure to maintain a normalized feminine appearance.

Sixteen years after her hysterectomy, Barbara was diagnosed with inflammatory breast cancer and had a mastectomy. A year after her diagnosis, she remains unsettled about her initial decision to avoid the prophylactic mastectomy. She said with an apologetic tone, "Now, I wish I'd taken that guy's advice. The mastectomy was still a hard thing to do. But, I'm sorry I didn't do it then and get phonies, although I can still get breast cancer post-mastectomy." Barbara acknowledges that a prophylactic procedure would not unequivocally prevent breast cancer. Because of the outcome, it is difficult for her to acknowledge that her reasons for rejecting the surgery may have been valid. She went on to say, "I just had too much, and I dismissed it." Given the gravity of Barbara's family history, the social pressure to take proactive medical action, and the depth of our discussion, it is hard for me to believe that Barbara would have made the decision without intensive consideration. Treatment and risk weighed heavily on the minds of all of the women I talked to. Yet making sense of one's prior decisions about treatment and risk sometimes requires people to reconstruct their personal histories.

The normalizing process involved in maintaining optimism requires a symbolic separation of the mind and body as she-roic survivors use rational systems of decision-making to manage their bodies, and engage feeling rules to manage their emotions.

Sixteen years earlier, Barbara was overwhelmed at the loss of her sister, her uterus, and her marriage. The rational decision to remove her breasts would have been emotionally devastating, and she was not willing to suppress her emotions at that point to make this decision. In her personal biography, however, Barbara concludes that she *should* have suppressed those emotions.

Because Barbara did not follow the rule of optimism 16 years earlier, she is well aware of it today. This is how she explained the optimism rule within her personal biography:

> I've had a good life. Even though it's been a tough life, it's been a good life, and a richly textured life. Very close friends, interesting experiences, and I want to live until I'm 75, but I know I won't. I'm more afraid of what I'm going to have to go through to die. I mean, there are times when I...I *shouldn't* say...I don't feel sorry for myself. There are times when I think..."I worked so hard, and I deserve more of this nice, happy marriage and good health and retirement than I'm gonna get... [My husband] deserves more...than he's gonna get.... I feel screwed." (emphasis added)

Barbara is aware that there are certain things she "shouldn't say." The rule of optimism demands that diagnosed women should *not* feel sorry for themselves, express fatalism, or "feel screwed." Instead, they should embody the she-ro who will "smile thru the tears" and "kick cancer's butt!" The mandate for positive thinking (Chapters 3 and 4) is represented in the war metaphor, personal cancer biographies, Lance Armstrong's sheer will to fight, Gilda Radner's humorous inspiration, and the numerous breast cancer sound bites and advertisements that illustrate smiling and hopeful survivors. Still, Barbara does not feel this way, even though she knows she should.

The disconnection between the feeling rules and women's actual feelings requires significant emotional work. If the work becomes too exhausting, some will aggressively reject the rule. Hearing Barbara's discontent, I asked her if she believed anything positive had come from her experience, and she replied:

> No! And, the next person who says to me, "Oh, but cancer makes you realize what's important in life, and learn what you really are, who you are"…I really knew who I was [and] what was important to me….I'm accelerating those things. I knew that an intimate relationship and friends were important. I didn't need cancer to learn those things. I would say that… what was the question?

Barbara was riled when I asked her about the potentially positive impact of her diagnosis. She immediately reacted and temporarily forgot the question. I repeated the question, and she replied:

> Life is precious and we take it for granted…I don't think anyone gets that message as much as when they know they're going to die sooner than they might have thought. We all know it's precious. And, I've gone back into not paying enough attention to that now that I'm feeling better. Because feeling

better makes you forget this cloud…I liked my life the way it *was* when I got sick. It's not that I was working at a horrible job and was going to quit, or I had a terrible mate or…that I made this great discovery when I really looked into my life… no, no, no, no, no!

Although I had not mentioned pink culture or survivor narratives, Barbara was aware of the stories of transcendence that dominate survivor imagery. She automatically identified the common themes, which Roslyn's story captured perfectly: horrible job, terrible mate, great discovery. As an act of defiance, Barbara defined her own sense of purpose and spoke emphatically that breast cancer was not responsible for it. Words like Barbara's would be characterized as negative in pink ribbon culture.

Breast cancer culture enforces the feeling rule of optimism either through the representation and positive reinforcement of normalization, hope, and transcendence, or by sanctioning negativity. Women have been "kicked out" of support groups and chat rooms for being unenthusiastic, angry, or depressed. Some women have told me that their doctors reprimanded them for having a negative attitude if they questioned medical authority or voiced concern about treatment. The upbeat climate of the culture requires whole-hearted optimism that is actively maintained with the explicit rejection of complaints. At the Avon 3-Day Breast Cancer Walk, the parade of pink will feature posters, buttons, T-shirts, and magnets with the "No Whining" symbol, a pink circle with a slash over the word "Whining."[6]

At the required introduction and safety sessions, participants view a 1-hour safety video that ends with the phrase, *no whining!* Walkers should understand clearly that there is no room for negativity in breast cancer survivorship.

Social support and a positive mental attitude can contribute to positive health outcomes, but they do not predict survival.[7] First, the dictum "no whining"—which often accompanies the adage "laughter is the best medicine"—is a cultural construct that makes optimism compulsory and omits the full range of emotional responses to cancer. I repeatedly heard women say that they "tried to be happy" when they felt differently. The emotional work to display optimism creates an added stressor, which can contribute to negative health outcomes.[8] Second, when the overemphasis on positive thinking places the burden of healing on the sick, it diverts attention from the social determinants of health—such as treatment modalities, access to care, support networks, and other factors known to influence healing processes. Third, the mandate for optimism creates a controlling image: the she-ro is a triumphant survivor. By definition she lives on, suggesting that the women who do not survive are not optimistic enough. This schism is hidden within the memorialization of those who died. Their names are written on billboards and T-shirts to pay tribute to their courage and the battle they fought. Their deaths cannot be incorporated into pink ribbon culture in any other way.

The pink ribbon culture typically overlooks these problems because optimism resonates with people on some level. Illnesses do have the potential to present people with opportunities for reflection and change that may have positive outcomes in various dimensions of their lives. Traumatic experiences may give rise to compassion and understanding in ways that promote social support and solidarity, especially among those who have had similarly difficult experiences. Barbara explains it in terms of empathy: "I think that [breast cancer] sharpens your sensitivity to other people's suffering, because you have suffered, and you know you will suffer." What Barbara and others reject is the overemphasis on transcendence, which encourages optimism to the point of encouraging women to conceal their distress based on the misguided belief that it will afford survival benefits.

FEELING RULE 2: SELFISHNESS

The diagnosis of breast cancer typically occurs over weeks or years, as women engage in breast self-examination, get regular mammograms, have biopsies, follow "watch and wait" protocols, and anticipate laboratory results. These prediagnostic events prepare women to spend considerable time thinking about themselves. After diagnosis, allopathic treatment processes require an extended self-focus as women make sense of the impact breast cancer has, and will have, on their lives and futures. Surgery, radiation, and chemotherapy are conventional treatments that typically entail multiple doctor visits, immersion in medical information, and conscientious decision-making. Treatments require time commitment for preparation, procedure, follow-up, mitigation of side effects, and recovery. Some women have reconstructive surgery, or undergo hormone and drug therapies to reduce their risk of recurrence. On average, the time frame from diagnosis through treatment is at least 1 year. Many of the women I interviewed were in treatment for several years, and some will be in treatment for the rest of their lives.

All of this thinking, feeling, and acting on behalf of one's health brings the self clearly into focus. The problem is that focusing on the self is not something women are supposed to do. The feeling rule of selfishness emphasizes social norms that stress women's nurturance, selflessness, and putting the needs of others first. *Feeling selfish* is a way for women to acknowledge this gender expectation. Diagnosed women contend with feelings of selfishness when they assess how they feel about putting their needs first, and what they do about how they feel. While the she-ro justifies selfishness as a rational and necessary form of self-care, feeling selfish is confessional, an admission of the gender violation that occurs when women shift their perspectives from putting the needs of others first to prioritizing their own needs.

She-roic Selfishness (i.e., Rational Coping Strategy)

Survivor narratives cast the she-ro as the archetypical protagonist in an epic tale of battle (Chapter 3). Character and plot are simple, recognizable, and portable. The she-ro integrates the valued masculine characteristics of strength, courage, and self-interestedness into her survivor identity as a combination of pink femininity and masculine power. The she-ro transcends breast cancer (and gender) with style and tenacity. The she-ro is not only an optimistic and informed medical consumer: she is also persuasive and assertive, expresses her needs to coworkers and family members, delegates responsibilities, and is successful in taking time for herself. While there is a correlation between leisure time and activities and improved mental and physical health,[9] the she-ro takes the modern ideal of individualism as the path to ultimate fulfillment to an extreme. Pink ribbon culture balances the heightened importance of self-interestedness through visions of sisterhood and unanimous support to the cause. It discounts the social roles and relational orientation central to the lives of women within families and other communities.

Women's paid work and unpaid family work typically involve taking care of others first and taking care of themselves second, third, fourth, or last. Early family socialization encourages boys to spend more time in leisure activities and girls to spend more time in household tasks, childcare, and other family work.[10] When internalized, these gendered patterns provide a normative reference point for individuals' expectations and entitlements. If nurturing is built into women's social roles when they are children and maintained into adulthood, then caring for others is likely to be an important part of women's identities. Nurturance may take on a selfless quality to the point that self-interest and femininity are seemingly incompatible. As the representative breast cancer survivor, the she-ro's sense of entitlement and self-interest is a role model for women who are not accustomed to putting themselves first.

The book *Breast Cancer? Let Me Check My Schedule* recognizes the challenges many women have fitting anything, including breast cancer, into their lives.[11] It describes the experiences of ten "remarkable" women who try—without skipping a beat—to balance their busy professional lives with the time they need to deal with breast cancer. The book reifies rational processes (time) as the primary way to manage body processes (breast cancer). The she-roes of the story resonate with women who need to balance work responsibilities with their personal lives, as one reviewer commented:[12]

> [The book] fits me to a "T." I too am a working woman complete with a little calendar that tells me when to have a headache. If it isn't penciled in, I don't have one. On April 23, 1992 under "Things to Do Today" I jotted down, "radical mastectomy, noon."

Although the details of this example may be applicable to a specific set of life circumstances for professional working women, the writer's sentiment is common among women whose lives revolve around meeting obligations and taking care of others.

When women are diagnosed with a chronic medical condition, they are less able to satisfy the gendered expectation of selflessness. Breast cancer forces women to interrupt their roles and regularly scheduled activities. This is not a desirable kind of "leisure," but it does impel women to opt out of their routines to reflect on their lives and priorities. Despite the difficulties of diagnosis and treatment, breast cancer provides a legitimized and compulsory reason for women to become self-interested. This is not always a welcome opportunity, especially for women who deeply value their caring roles. Many women, however, do appreciate the chance to consider their personal needs and interests. Fifty-four-year-old Mary explained that chemotherapy treatment enabled her to take time for herself:

> All my life I never took the time for me…For those six months [during chemotherapy] I was basically by myself…I wasn't around people because I couldn't be…[I was] on antibiotics… Other than [immediate family], I did not see people…There was a blessing in that…It forced me to be with me.

Mary's life circumstances had encouraged her to suppress her needs and interests to take on nurturing and service roles in her private and public life. Mary's experience sheds light on why breast cancer might be called a "blessing" for women who spend the bulk of their time in imbalanced care work situations.

When people do something that breaks with convention, they have to account for their behavior.[13] Women who are nurturing and empathetic behave consistently with traditional gender role expectations, and there is no explanation required. However, selflessness is a social expectation that chronic illness typically forces women to breach. In this case, women must account for their actions, reframing selfishness as a rational coping strategy. Forty-eight-year-old Amy said: "I don't consider myself selfish in the point that I look after myself. I consider myself smart to look after myself." Amy casts her behavior in masculine terms, separating rationality (traditionally associated with the masculine) from emotionality (traditionally associated with the feminine). Rationality confers social value to Amy's transgressive behavior.

Amy went on to say, however, "but, I don't always look after myself first." To affirm her femininity, Amy offers assurances that she does not *always* look after herself *first*. To do so would suggest a socially unacceptable level of self-interest for a woman.

As an established social space, pink ribbon culture encourages women to acknowledge their survivor status, participate in sensitizing breast cancer activities, and support other diagnosed women. As women become part of established survivor networks, there is support for reframing self-interest from a traditionally feminine characterization (selfishness) to a she-roic interpretation (rational coping strategy necessary for health). Forty-three-year-old Linda talked about how striving to be the "best mother, best worker, and perfectionist to boot" left her with little time to "sit with [her] feelings." When breast cancer compelled Linda to consider her needs first, she had to "cut [herself] some slack." This meant renegotiating her social roles and responsibilities, providing justification, and adjusting her personal and social expectations. Linda relied heavily on pink ribbon culture and her survivor status to do this. Even though she was not initially "into wearing pink ribbons," she described how her participation in, and support for, "the cause" emerged spontaneously:

> It seems to me that you automatically get these roles even if you're not…looking for them!! I have already been called upon to provide support for two other women…When my new boss discovered that I was a breast cancer survivor, she decided we should all participate in the Avon 3-Day walk for breast cancer…now I'm raising money for the walk and going to walk 60 miles in 3 days in August…I'm really glad [my boss] said "we have to do this" because it has caused me to get out and exercise… I'm a happier person who eats better and takes better care of herself than I was before.

Linda's narrative demonstrates how pink ribbon culture is organized to promote automatic support for the cause and participation in the culture. First, the culture promotes a sisterhood of survivorship through obligatory voluntarism. Second, the activities define social support in terms of fundraising and mass public involvement in symbolic action. Third, an underlying belief that sustains these actions is that survivor participation in pink ribbon culture is transformative, playing a vital role in helping diagnosed women to maintain their physical and mental health.

The feeling rule of selfishness encourages self-discipline as women assess their feelings and validate their behavior. As women foster self-interest as a rational coping strategy, the relationship between survivorship and feminine identity surfaces.

Diagnosed women who participate in pink ribbon culture and/ or identify with she-roic standards are able to engage in a mode of survivorship that results in the recontextualization of selfishness (as a gender transgression) into a socially acceptable coping strategy. Self-interest is empowering to some women; for others, it is shameful or impossible.

Selfishness as Confessional

Breast cancer shapes how diagnosed women look at their lives and at themselves, both as women and as survivors. As I heard repeatedly, the illness experience can shift women's perspectives about what is important, how to spend time, the meaning of personal relationships, opinions about the medical system, views about "the cause" and existing systems of social support, and feelings about how to cope. With consistency, the women I interviewed believed that a self-focused stance was necessary and justified. When a self-interested perspective necessitated changes in social interaction or was disruptive to others, the feeling rule of selfishness provided an account for women's feelings and behavior. If women did not uphold self-interestedness as a rational approach to breast cancer as the she-ro prescribes, they tended to characterize it as an affront to traditional femininity—as selfishness. The breast cancer biography that follows echoes many diagnosed women who regularly dealt with feelings of selfishness. For these women, putting their needs first contributed to social stigma rather than empowerment.

Alice was diagnosed with breast cancer at age 52. She worked as a customer service agent, was married, had three grown children, and had no history of the disease in her family. Prior to her diagnosis, Alice was in good general health. She went to the same doctor for 15 years for routine annual checkups and started having regular mammograms every other year beginning at age 45. Prior to her diagnosis, Alice had no symptoms and no palpable masses. In 1992, Alice had an annual gynecological examination that included a clinical breast examination and a routine mammogram. The clinical examination revealed nothing. Three days later, the doctor called Alice to tell her that the mammogram showed a large mass. After meeting with her doctor, she scheduled a lumpectomy to remove and biopsy the mass. During the procedure, the surgeon found three masses instead of one. The surgeon removed all of them, along with five lymph nodes. The biopsy revealed that the masses and the lymph nodes contained breast cancer cells, and Alice was diagnosed with stage 4 invasive breast cancer.

The type of invasive breast cancer that Alice had was infiltrating lobular carcinoma, which represents about 10 to 15 percent of invasive breast cancers. Infiltrating lobular carcinoma begins in the milk-producing glands, invades the breast's fatty tissue, and has the potential to spread elsewhere in the body. It is often difficult to detect by physical examination or by mammography, which explains why Alice's breast cancer was not diagnosed despite routine mammography screening and clinical examination. To treat her stage 4 breast cancer, Alice had a mastectomy,

8 months of chemotherapy, and 4 years of adjuvant drug therapy with tamoxifen, a drug designed to slow or stop the growth
of lingering cancer cells of a certain type of cancer that is hor-
mone-sensitive. At the time of our interview, Alice told me she
was lucky to be in the 11 percent of women with a stage 4 diagnosis who are still alive at 7 years after diagnosis. The lack of
accurate information about staging, breast cancer types, and the
limitations of early detection contribute to societal and individual misunderstanding about how to deal with breast cancer.
It certainly added to Alice's confusion about why her breast
cancer was found so "late."

Alice's treatment had a profound impact on her everyday life
for the 5-year period following her diagnosis. For 3 months after
the mastectomy, she could not reach over her head or lift a bag
of groceries and had pain in her arm from the removal of lymph
nodes. She suffered from frequent infections that required regular ultrasounds and multiple rounds of antibiotics, and she
experienced side effects from tamoxifen. Alice concluded that
tamoxifen-induced hormonal imbalances were the cause of her
intense emotional difficulties, saying:

> [Tamoxifen]… [takes] you through your menopause again,
> with the hot flashes and everything like that. They say there's
> no mental effect, but I was terrible. I was just crazy for four
> years, screaming at my husband, crying for…days at a time…
> I had to stay home from work one day because I was crying
> all day…I thought I was going crazy.

Hormonal imbalances from tamoxifen may or may not have been the main source of Alice's emotional difficulties. The National Cancer Institute has not documented a "mental effect" as a result of tamoxifen, though memory changes have been associated with chemotherapy, which Alice also endured. The documented side effects of tamoxifen range from blood clots, strokes, uterine cancer, and cataracts to symptoms comparable to menopause such as hot flashes, headaches, fatigue, nausea, vaginal discharge, and irregular menstruation.[14] Any of these side effects could contribute to emotional distress. Alice's cancer biography alludes to additional sources of stress that many women experience after diagnosis, which involve changes in family and other personal relationships.

Families play a crucial role in providing care and social support for family members with serious illnesses.[15] There is a social expectation that families should fill the gaps in support that are left by inadequate social institutions, and that they should do so successfully and without hesitation. When women share their diagnosis story, discussions of supportive family relationships usually come first. Positive family relationships go along with feeling optimistic about one's life and future. Discussions of unsupportive family relationships typically surface later, when women discuss breast cancer as a disruption to family life and their role in the family system. Alice's son never talked to her about her illness experience, though she was told by his girlfriend that he was very upset for the 2 weeks following his mother's diagnosis. Alice's oldest daughter was angry with her mother for getting sick. Alice's youngest daughter made demands on her father to take care of Alice. And Alice's husband did not like his wife's post-treatment body or attitude. These family dynamics bothered Alice, and she said many times throughout our conversation that she was "depressed" about them. At the same time, Alice was resigned to what she believed was an uncompromising situation. She said, "I mean, what are you supposed to do?"

To get on, Alice did what many people do: she used comparative rationalizations that would enable her to accept her circumstances. In explaining her children's responses she said, "The kids aren't going to do much for you, even though you think they will...They have their own lives." To explain her husband's response, she said, "There are worse things [my husband] could have done...he's not going to leave me [at his age]." Many women used an "It could have been worse" ledger to account for changes in their family relationships after diagnosis. In using "It could have been worse" to explain family disruption, women recognized that their illness experiences changed how accessible they were to their families. They were no longer selfless. If diagnosed women were not able to claim entitlement to self-interestedness, they felt stigmatized by it. Feeling selfish is a way to confess to the gender violation and accept the consequences.

Women are supposed to be selfless, putting the needs of others (especially family) before their own. Any break from this expectation requires acknowledgement. Many women accounted for their shift in perspective and behavior in terms of an obligatory coping response. But instead of determining self-interestedness to be rational, they called it selfish. Alice explains that putting her needs first was essential, selfish, and incompatible with family responsibilities:

When you get breast cancer you have to think more about yourself. I thought more of myself than the family, the husband, or the kids…You have to become selfish…Before, I couldn't think about myself at all, because I had to take care of my kids and my family. If they needed something, they came first. After breast cancer, I had to turn to myself.[16]

Alice's statement conveys the difficulty many women have putting themselves first. She went on to explain that selfishness was multidimensional, including time, energy, money, and self-fulfilling choices. Because Alice did not feel entitled to these things, she viewed them as selfish.

Responding to breast cancer requires concentrated effort and self-focus that forces women to break with their daily routines and pay attention to their needs. The circumstances of women's lives and illness experiences vary in terms of diagnosis, prognosis, doctor–patient interactions, satisfaction with treatment, insurance coverage, finances, family dynamics, work situations, and support networks. Yet, with great regularity, diagnosed women engage the feeling rule of selfishness to manage the transgression of self-investment. The simultaneous acknowledgement and defense of selfishness illustrates the tension between gender expectations for women's selflessness and she-roic expectations for women's rational self-interestedness. Pink ribbon culture promotes the latter interpretation, with a strong focus on the empowered role of the survivor. Confessional selfishness and guilt work in similar ways; as internalized stigma.

FEELING RULE 3: GUILT

Despite social consensus that breast cancer is a good cause and survivorship a valued status, many diagnosed women continue to face social stigma associated with breast cancer as (a) failure to present oneself adequately as a she-ro, (b) embodied social stigma, or (c) burden to families and others. As with the first two feeling rules, guilt revolves around normative expectations related to gender and pink ribbon culture. Diagnosed women who embody the she-ro by embracing optimism and reframing selfishness as a rational coping strategy are not supposed to feel guilt. On the contrary, failing to present oneself as a she-ro undermines pink ribbon culture and is guilt-inducing. If the aesthetic approach to normalization is not successful, breast cancer continues to be a threat to bodily integrity and, therefore, femininity. In this situation women may feel guilty about having breast cancer, and they may feel responsible for bringing it on themselves. Also, women who are the principal providers of care and concern for others are likely to feel guilty if they are unable to maintain these requirements after diagnosis.

The Inadequate She-ro

As diagnosed women negotiate the feeling rules of optimism, selfishness, and guilt, the characteristics of the she-ro play an important role. Some women feel stigmatized or blameworthy for not being optimistic *enough*, empowered *enough*, and she-roic *enough*. Although some women consciously reject she-roic standards of survivorship and instead participate in subaltern processes and/or communities, the failure to present oneself in accord with the accepted culture can lead to social sanctions and feelings of guilt. In particular, women with invasive, advanced, or recurring breast cancers do not fit easily into the pink mold. Angie's story speaks to the uneasy relationship that these women are likely to have with the pink mainstream.

At age 48, Angie was diagnosed with infiltrating ductal carcinoma, which is the most common type of invasive breast cancer and accounts for 80 percent of malignancies. Unlike most diagnosed women (about 90 percent) who do *not* have a family history of breast cancer,[17] Angie's mother and aunt died from the disease. At the time of Angie's diagnosis, the cancer was at stage 4; it had already spread to other organs of the body. As with Alice—who had been diagnosed at stage 4 but with a different type of invasive breast cancer—Angie found her tumor between routine screenings and regular clinical examinations. Because Angie's mother had died from the disease, she already knew that early detection was a misnomer for all breast cancers. Yet Angie still dealt with the mythology surrounding early detection. Although there is a general consensus that women at later stages of diagnosis are less likely to survive long term, the increased prevalence and visibility of early-stage (especially stage 0) breast cancers creates a triumphant portrait of survivorship.

There is a general impression that the treatment of early breast cancer is now successful and relatively short-lived. There may be nausea, vomiting, hair loss, fatigue, and surgical procedures, but the focus on improved survival rates justifies any disruptions, difficulties, or side effects. Recognizing this trend, Angie said, "[breast cancer] is almost like old hat for people." Yet for Angie and the 40 percent of diagnosed women who are *not* in the "early stage" category, treatment is not easy, and it may last for the rest of their lives. Angie said, "I'm HER-2/neu positive.[18] That means my own body is feeding [the cancer] at a more rapid rate... For me, it's never gonna be over." Although Angie undergoes regular treatment, she knows that on average only about 20 percent of women with stage 4 breast cancer live for 5 years.[19] At the time of our interview, Angie had already survived 4 years, and she was not confident that she would live until the 5-year mark.

Angie's perspective about her prognosis was based on informed and rational assessment. Her non-optimistic tone, coupled with the visible effects of ongoing treatment, made others feel "uncomfortable." In a cancer culture where hope is the touchstone of survivorship, it can be difficult for people to acknowledge when diagnosed persons do not feel good or have good prospects for long-term survival. Women at later stages told me about numerous situations when family, friends, neighbors, and other survivors did not want to acknowledge their realities. This left the women feeling isolated and unsupported, and it also called into question the authenticity of their illness experience. Angie described it this way:

> This is not the breast cancer story people want to hear….but, it's real. It's happening. It's happening to me…I was with some people who were all talking about this… [other] family who was having some problems. Not one of them said, "How are you doing, Angie? How are things going for you?" I'm in treatment every week… I'm not really trying for attention, but this is the reality of my life and they're not comfortable with it…I was upset that they couldn't even acknowledge something I was going through. And, it made me feel guilty for even feeling upset.

Angie realizes that her situation is distressing to others, but she is troubled that she cannot share her experiences openly and honestly. With a semblance of optimism, she tries not to "feel sorry for [her]self." Angie understands that there is a proper breast cancer story, one that does not apply to her. Angie's statement that she was "not trying for attention" is an acknowledgement that presenting oneself outside of the breast cancer norm automatically draws attention. Angie's lived experience is different from the norms that dominate pink culture and therefore is a social breach. Based on the candor of her previous statements, it seems that Angie believes she has a right to be upset, yet she still feels guilty.

Embodied Social Stigma

Women who do not live up to the expectations of pink culture face an ongoing stigma. In addition, women who believed they had made the wrong decisions for the wrong reasons earlier in their lives often felt responsible for causing their breast cancer. This sense of personal responsibility confers greater social force to the feeling rules. The stigma associated with breast cancer as a physical and social threat is sometimes internalized in women's feelings about their post-treatment bodies or about having breast cancer in the first place.

In addition to dealing with physical and emotional side effects of breast cancer treatment, diagnosed women come to terms with their feelings about having a body that does not conform to normative feminine expectations. The aesthetic approach to normalization discussed in Chapter 2 focuses on outward appearance following breast cancer treatment for this reason. I regularly heard women's concerns about self-image and social interactions that reinforced feelings of shame. Some of these women's stories were embarrassing or comical, such as the lopsided wig or the prosthesis that floated out of a woman's swimsuit at a public pool. Most clothing, including swimsuits, is not made for one-breasted women. Other social interactions were hurtful, and all of them reinforced women's outsider status based on having a nonconforming body.

Alice, for example, was an avid swimmer. After her mastectomy, she used a prosthesis in her swimsuit and moved it to her bra after showering. One day she forgot it, and others in the locker room took notice:

> Even though the shirt was baggy...They were looking...
> I could hear them saying, "Do you see her? She doesn't have
> a..." It's a shock to them to see somebody they don't consider
> normal...what are you supposed to do? Just be fat and be old?

Alice describes herself and her body in self-deprecating ways, but she was embarrassed. She went on to justify the reaction, saying, "It's kind of grotesque...it's not like you've lost half of your face, and you have burns or something. There are a lot of things in life that are a lot worse than that... I'm just flat on one side." Many women used comparative rationalizations to accept the stigma of their post-treatment body.

Part of bodily acceptance involves the relationship between looking good and feeling better. Certainly, the American Cancer Society's "Look Good, Feel Better" program actively promotes this message when it assists women with wigs, prosthetics, and cosmetics following treatment. Alice uses this belief to mitigate the social stigma of her post-treatment body. She said, "I used to be a thin thing, and now I'm not... [But] you can't expect to fit into a [size] 7 when you wear a [size] 12. So you buy nice 12s, and then you look better." The extent to which aesthetic strategies alter self-image can be limited. Despite wearing a prosthesis or buying new clothes, Alice still uses the word *grotesque* to describe her body, and she has reinforcement for this belief. She said, "[My husband] thinks it is very grotesque looking. It does bother him a lot. I think my weight gain [after treatment] bothered him even more." Alice balances her husband's opinion of her physical appearance, saying, "I still keep insisting [to my husband], if you look at girls I went to school with, their bellies are down to here. I'm not that bad. I wear a 12, but it's not so bad. And, he doesn't wear 28s any more either. It's 36s. But, yeah, it's depressing."

Embodied social stigma is also visible in women's feelings of personal responsibility for getting breast cancer in the first place. Even though the causes of breast cancer are not known, many diagnosed women feel potentially at fault for causing their own breast cancer. Scientists have uncovered some of the risk factors associated with breast cancer (such as age, reproductive factors, inherited genetic mutations, postmenopausal obesity, hormone replacement therapy, alcohol consumption, and previous history of endometrial, ovarian, or colon cancer). Less than 30 percent of diagnosed women have any of these known risk factors, creating uncertainty about causation.[20] Without certainty, many women ask the question: "What did *I* do to cause this?" Whether it was perceived to be punishment from God or the consequence of poor lifestyle choices, the quest for cause was a quest for blame.

Roslyn's initial reaction to her diagnosis was that it was punishment for leaving her husband. After she concluded that marital dissolution was not the likely cause, she spent 2 years searching for what was. Roslyn described what she calls her "big study":

After my diagnosis, my big study was, "How did I get it? What did I do to cause this?" And [the doctors] said, "You'll probably never know…" I was not comfortable with that answer. I had done so much research trying to find out why… what did I do to cause it? Was it taking birth control pills when I was younger? I was never on hormones. Was it environmental? I run every day…Was it that pounding that did it? Was it the cars?…I spent two years trying to figure out how this could have happened when it wasn't in my family…and I could not move forward…now I realize I may never know.[21]

Scrutinizing one's lifestyle and decisions is a common response to a breast cancer diagnosis, particularly within a social context that emphasizes individualism and personal responsibility. When women are unable to pinpoint a cause, they must adjust to the uncertainty of not knowing what caused their breast cancer. Roslyn eventually conceded, following the advice of a doctor who told her to "get past this and think about the future." Although diagnosed women may be absolved of the guilt associated with *causing* their breast cancer, they still contend with feeling guilty about *having* breast cancer.

Family Disruption

Barbara said it plainly, "The fact that I have cancer makes me feel guilty." With great regularity the guilt associated with having cancer reflected women's concerns about the emotional stress and disruption that it caused in their families. Women's roles in the family typically revolve around "caring for" and "caring about" other family members. Any disruption to this complex network of caring and concern necessarily affects family roles and expectations. In addition to feeling a sense of loss about being unable to fully maintain their regular roles and meet expectations, many women also felt guilty about it. The types of things women would feel guilty about were far-ranging, from marital disruption to causing worry in others to burdening their children to seemingly trivial incidents.

Breast cancer symbolizes the inability of diagnosed women to protect the people they care about from difficulty and discomfort. Barbara's guilt was related to what she described as "the misery [she] brought into [her] marriage." When discussing her non-optimistic feelings about breast cancer earlier in this chapter, Barbara shared that she and her husband had earned a good life and happy marriage, and that breast cancer was going to take this privilege from them. Since she was the one diagnosed, Barbara took ownership for the difficulty and suffering that she perceived *her* breast cancer was causing in *her* marriage. Such personal responsibility does not take into account that the causes of breast cancer are not known, that treatment responses are largely outside of one's control, or that her husband plays a role in the marriage. But it does give Barbara the tools to feel guilty. To protect her husband from further burden and emotional strife, she tried to keep her fear, anxiety, and pain to herself. Guilt enables women to re-identify with feminine selflessness when the conditions of their lives prevent them from fully engaging in their nurturing roles.

At the time of our interview—4 years after her diagnosis—Roslyn regretted that her adult children were present when she received her diagnosis. She had explicitly told them not to go to the doctor's office, but they "showed up anyway." The memory of her daughter's face when she heard the diagnosis played an important role in Roslyn's emotion work. She said,

> I remember looking...at my daughter...if I could have taken back his words...the look on her face, I will never forget. That's my one regret...that she was there, and she did hear it...and I could not...I wanted to shield her from the abrupt, "You have breast cancer."

It did not matter that neither the situation nor the diagnosis was within Roslyn's locus of control: the diagnosis incident compromised Roslyn's ability as a mother to protect her child from distress. Roslyn's feelings of remorse from this single occurrence would later affect decisions about how much to handle on her own, and how much she should rely on others for support.

When care work is deeply embedded in women's roles and identities, any incident that compromises women's abilities to express nurturance and love can initiate feelings of guilt. Fifty-five-year-old Vivien describes a food-related episode with her stepson:

> I've always made [my stepchildren] cookies...They are in their thirties now, and they still want those cookies. [My stepson] hadn't been home for a few years...and I still wasn't really into my good mode...and he went to the cookie jar. It was empty. I said, "I couldn't do it."...and he was like, "Okay." He was trying to be understanding, but he really wanted those cookies...and I felt so guilty.[22]

Vivien's guilt involves the management of others' perceptions, and the internalization of stigma related to her role in the family. Although she believed she was justified in taking her health into account, she blames herself for disappointing her stepson.

The tension between taking care of herself and taking care of others was visible as Vivien continued to explain her guilt:

> I said, "Why am I feeling guilty?" I couldn't do them, and I didn't do them, and that was that. And I said, "When I see him, I'll bring him some cookies." But it was something that normally I would have just gotten out of bed if I was sick and made those cookies for him. But I just don't do those things anymore.[23]

After having breast cancer, Vivien's actions deviated from what had been normal in her family. The guilt that comes from this deviation is a reflection of internalized stigma. Even though Vivien was somewhat defiant about her right to put herself and her health first, she regretted not being able to set her needs aside. She assuages her guilt by holding out the promise of normative behavior in the future.

CONCLUSION

When facing breast cancer, social context provides a benchmark for evaluating one's emotions and responses. The feeling rules of survivorship are the guidelines that enable diagnosed women to asses how they "should" or "should not" feel about breast cancer. These conventions of feeling provide an explanatory framework that exerts social force on women's decisions, coping strategies, interactions with others, and sense of self. Women's personal histories illuminate these feeling rules, and the emotional work required to manage them, within their cancer biographies. By analyzing the patterns of commonality and difference in women's behaviors, coping mechanisms, and cultural repertoires as women describe them in their narratives, we see how social and cultural expectations become embedded within people's personal lives and how social rules are often simultaneous and mutually reinforcing.

Optimism, selfishness, and guilt are conventions of feeling that integrate social expectations prevalent within pink ribbon culture and the broader gender system:

- **Optimism**: Hope, faith, transcendence, and the power of positive thinking intersect with pink femininity and pink ribbon culture to construct she-roic optimism for breast cancer survivors. The she-ro displays feminine empowerment, an aesthetic approach to normalization, and the suppression of negativity. If women choose to uphold this standard, they must restrain feelings of anxiety, depression, concern, or pain.

- **Selfishness**: In accord with the she-ro model, selfishness can be reframed as self-interestedness, a rational form of coping; or feeling selfish is a way to acknowledge women's violations of gender expectations that call for women's selflessness.

- **Guilt**: May occur when diagnosed women do not present themselves according to she-roic standards, are self-conscious about changes to their bodies, or are concerned that their diagnosis causes worry and disruption in their families.

The stories told in this chapter help us to understand how elements of social context influence the perspectives and experiences of women diagnosed with breast cancer. After learning the rules to become a breast cancer survivor and using these rules to construct a personal cancer biography, women then negotiate with others to maintain a coherent sense of self. The feeling rules of breast cancer survivorship empower and constrain throughout the breast cancer experience and within women's particular circumstances. In Chapter 7, I look at how the rules contribute to a "balancing act" as women try to carve out their own mode of survivorship and establish equilibrium between their needs and the needs of others.

NOTES

1. A. Hochschild, *The Managed Heart: The Commercialization of Human Feeling* (Berkeley: University of California Press, 2003), 7.

2. E. Lang, K. S. Berbaum, & S. K. Lutgendorf, et al., "Large-Core Breast Biopsy: Abnormal Salivary Cortisol Profiles Associated with Uncertainty…" *Radiology* 250 (2009): 631-7.

3. M. Bury, "Chronic Illness as Biographical Disruption," *Sociology of Health and Illness* 4, no. 2 (1982): 167-82.

4. A. Hochschild, "Emotion Work, Feeling Rules, and Social Structure," *American Journal of Sociology* 85, no. 3 (1979): 551-75.

5. "Obsessed with Breasts Public Awareness Campaign," Breast Cancer Fund, http://www.breastcancerfund.org/site/pp.asp?c=kwKXLdPaE&b=83016.

6. Participants can purchase the "No Whining" breast cancer line at http://www.cafepress.com/medtees/907177: "Humorous and Thoughtful Apparel and Merchandise for the Irreverent Patient."

7. A. Steptoe & A. Appels, eds., *Stress, Personal Controls and Health* (Chichester, England: Wiley, 1989); L. F. Berkman, T. Glass, I. Brissette, & T. E. Seeman, "From Social Integration to Health: Durkheim in the New Millennium," *Social Science and Medicine* 51 (2000): 843-57; D. Blane, E. Brunner, & R. Wilkinson, eds., *Health and Social Organization: Towards a Health Policy for the 21st Century* (London: Routledge, 1996); J. Coyne, T. Pajak, J. Harris, A. Konski, B. Movsas, K. Ang, D.W. Bruner, et al., "Emotional Well-Being Does Not Predict Survival in Head and Neck Cancer Patients," *Cancer* 110 (October 22, 2007): 2568-75; M. Petticrew, "Influence of Psychological Coping on Survival and Recurrence in People with Cancer: Systematic Review," *British Medical Journal* 325 (November 7, 2002): 1066-9.

8. Petticrew, "Influence of Psychological Coping on Survival and Recurrence in People with Cancer: Systematic Review."

9. C. Goodwin & R. P. Hill, "Commitment to Physical Fitness: Commercial Influences on Long-Term Healthy Consumer Behaviors," *Social Marketing Quarterly* 4 (Spring 1998): 68-83; K. A. Henderson, "The Meaning of Leisure for Women: An Integrative Review of the Research," *Journal of Leisure Research* 22, no. 3 (1990): 228-43; K. A. Henderson &

D. M. Bialeschki, "A Sense of Entitlement to Leisure as Constraint and Empowerment for Women," *Leisure Sciences* 13, no. 1 (1991): 51-66.

10. V. McGann & J. Steil, "The Sense of Entitlement: Implications for Gender Equality and Psychological Well-Being," in *Handbook of Girls' and Women's Psychological Health: Gender and Well-Being Across the Life Span,* eds. J. Worell & C. Goodheart (New York: Oxford University Press, 2005), 175-82; B. Major, "From Social Inequality to Personal Entitlement: The Role of Social Comparisons, Legitimacy Appraisals, and Group Membership," in *Advances in Experimental Social Psychology,* ed. M. Zanna (San Diego: Academic Press, 1994), 293-355.

11. P. McCarthy & J. Loren, *Breast Cancer? Let Me Check My Schedule!: Ten Remarkable Women Meet the Challenge of Fitting Breast Cancer Into Their Very Busy Lives* (Boulder, CO: Westview Press, 1997).

12. B. Gay, review of *Breast Cancer? Let Me Check My Schedule!: Ten Remarkable Women Meet the Challenge of Fitting Breast Cancer Into Their Very Busy Lives,* by P. McCarthy & J. Loren, Amazon.com, http://www.amazon.com/Breast-Cancer-Let-Check-Schedule/dp/0813334314.

13. M. B. Scott & S. Lyman, "Accounts," *American Sociological Review* 33 (1968): 46062; S. Lyman & M. B. Scott, *A Sociology of the Absurd* (New York: Appleton-Century Crofts, 1970).

14. "Tamoxifen: Questions and Answers," National Cancer Institute Fact Sheet, http://www.cancer.gov/cancertopics/factsheet/therapy/tamoxifen.

15. D. Karp, *The Burden of Sympathy: How Families Cope with Mental Illness* (New York: Oxford University Press, 2001); D. Paterniti & K. Charmaz, *Health, Illness, and Healing: Society, Social Context, and Self* (Los Angeles: Roxbury, 1999); P. Reynolds, S. Hurley, M. Torres, et al., "Use of Coping Strategies and Breast Cancer Survival: Results from the Black/White Cancer Survival Study," *American Journal of Epidemiology* 152 (2000): 940-9.

16. G. Sulik, "On the Receiving End: Women, Caring, and Breast Cancer," *Qualitative Sociology* 30, no. 3 (2007): 305.

17. M. Kriege, C. T. M. Brekelmans, C. Boetes, et al., "Efficacy of MRI and Mammography for Breast-Cancer Screening in Women with a Familial or Genetic Predisposition," *New England Journal of Medicine* 351, no. 5 (2004): 427-37.

18. HER-2/neu is an example of one of the dominant oncogenes that contribute to cancer that is frequently overexpressed. HER-2/neu-positive tumors tend to be more aggressive. S. M. Love with K. Lindsey, *Dr. Susan Love's Breast Book* (New York: Addison-Wesley, 2005), 334.

19. *Medline Plus Encyclopedia,* s.v. "Breast Cancer," http://www.nlm.nih.gov/MEDLINEPLUS/ency/article/000913.htm (accessed October 1, 2009).

20. B. S. Hulka & A. T. Stark, "Breast Cancer: Cause and Prevention," *Lancet* 346 (1995): 883-7; S. M. Love with K. Lindsey, *Dr. Susan Love's Breast Book*; S. A. Smith-Warner, D. Spiegelman, & S. S. Yaun, "Alcohol and Breast Cancer in Women: A Pooled Analysis of Cohort Studies," *Journal of the American Medical Association* 279, no. 7 (1998): 535-40.

21. See G. Sulik, G. A. Sulik, & A. Eich-Krohm, "No Longer a Patient: The Social Construction of the Medical Consumer," in *Patients, Consumers and Civil Society*, ed. S. Chambre & M. Goldner, vol. 10 in *Advances in Medical Sociology* (Bingley, UK: Emerald Group, 2008), 3-28.

22. Sulik, "On the Receiving End," 305.

23. *Ibid.*

SEVEN

The Balancing Act

O n a December evening before the holidays, 51-year-old Sarah received a telephone call. She said, "I remember the chilling feeling…when the surgeon told me that…there were breast cancer cells. It was like somebody pulled down a shade. It was that dramatic…a feeling of aloneness, of isolation… It didn't go away…Being told I had breast cancer, just made me feel alone." The loneliness Sarah describes continued well into her treatment and aftercare. Although she eventually developed ways to deal with her feelings and the physical and logistical challenges that resulted from breast cancer, she continues to feel isolation whenever she remembers her experience or thinks about the future. What's more, she is isolated from pink ribbon culture. Sarah is not a member of the united front of survivors who are draped in pink, enthusiastically supporting one another, selflessly organized, and optimistically calling attention to the need for awareness, research, and funding in the fight against breast cancer. The hope, courage, and inspiration at the center of this culture are inaccessible to Sarah. As a result, she and many other breast cancer survivors develop their own ways of coping, reminding us that despite mass public attention to the cause of breast cancer, the illness is a very lonely place to be.

The early breast cancer movement established support programs to mitigate the isolation that typically accompanies cancer diagnosis and treatment. Today, many support groups, education programs, and community-building events are built on the idea that when people who have similar life experiences share those experiences, solidarity emerges, support systems form, and feelings of inclusion alleviate feelings of isolation. Pink ribbon culture developed from this social history. Yet, today's breast cancer culture dictates the terms of women's shared experience in ways that marginalize those who do not passionately participate and cheerfully comply with the culture's rules of survivorship. There is no room for lackluster support, contemplation of scientific controversies, inquiry into conflicts of interest between breast cancer advocacy and the cancer industry, alternative ways of coping that do not involve pink consumption, or public health strategies that do not rely on the mass proliferation of screening programs. Promoting the affirming message that all breast cancer survivors are equal sisters in a community of survivorship, pink ribbon culture has succeeded in spreading the message that its cultural leaders have figured out how best to fight the war on breast cancer, while burgeoning community outreach programs uphold an assumption that the culture itself provides diagnosed women with abundant pathways for care and social support.

Pink ribbon culture thrives. Yet for many women, the war is a lost cause and social support wanes. Barbara Ehrenreich and Samantha King point out that the culture surrounding breast cancer survivorship operates tyrannically, using cheerfulness as a form of social control to normalize and depoliticize the disease.[1] A positive attitude and self-presentation encourage pink consumption and broad participation in the culture while simultaneously suppressing realities that do not fit the pink mold. Women are left with two choices: Become a member of the sisterhood, or fend for yourself. As diagnosed women confront pink ribbon culture, they quickly learn the criteria for becoming full-fledged members. The culture relies on the regular voluntary participation of well-meaning and enthusiastic survivors to run support groups, participate in education and advocacy programs, raise funds, and rally widespread support for, and participation in, the cause. Such volunteerism encourages diagnosed women to put the needs of others first (especially other survivors), while using the rhetoric of personal empowerment within the context of medical consumerism and the breast cancer brand. When the quintessential she-ro of pink ribbon culture deals with breast cancer, she claims her status as a survivor, takes control, remains positive, manages difficulty, gains respect and admiration from those around her, and, with the help of modern medicine, beats the disease. Popular she-ro imagery valorizes optimism, camaraderie, courage, and women's selflessness. As the numerous advertisements suggest, if a diagnosed woman can walk a 5-kilometer race without "whining" to fight the war on breast cancer, anyone can.

Many diagnosed women participate in pink ribbon culture for a time and feel empowered doing so. However, the widely distributed imagery of the 1.3 million participants in the annual Komen Race for the Cure series and the tens of thousands of women who participate in the Avon walks, donning smiling faces and pink paraphernalia, do not reflect the illness experiences of the 210 million women in the United States who are currently living with breast cancer. Women whose diagnoses, personal dispositions, and life circumstances encourage alternative ways of responding to breast cancer fall outside of the pink mainstream. Public spectacle obscures how these women face stigma, isolation, limited care, and a lack of social support. As the previous chapter discussed, women are sometimes so accustomed to paying attention to the needs of others and responding to those needs that it can be difficult for them to break from this pattern when the roles are reversed. The she-ro of pink ribbon culture encourages women to become optimistic medical consumers and empowered participants in the sisterhood of survivorship, revising social roles and expectations, if necessary, to do so. The she-roic model incorporates gender expectations into pink femininity (feminine appearance, conciliatory behavior, emotional sensitivity, social restraint, and feminine accoutrements), but it does not take into account the contexts of women's everyday lives.

There are two attitudes in American society that would kindle the belief that women diagnosed with breast cancer should get support, while reducing the efficacy and availability of that support. First, breast cancer advocacy has institutionalized the idea of social support for diagnosed women, while pink ribbon culture has limited social support to practices within the sisterhood. Second, women in families regularly fill gaps in support for family members who are ill or in crisis. When women get sick, who takes care of them? Both of these situations create social conditions that encourage women to place the needs and wants of others (breast cancer survivors or family members) before their own. In turn, many diagnosed women are responsible for taking care of themselves, without much support.

TAKING CARE OF MYSELF

Pink ribbon culture promotes the normalization of breast cancer while simultaneously systematizing the availability of support. The message is that the diagnosed are not alone, and that there are mechanisms in place to provide emotional and practical support. Underlying this message is an assumption that only "survivors" who have "been through it" can serve this function. The isolation associated with breast cancer is so strong that many women believe no one outside of the survivor circle has the capacity to understand and feel what they are feeling. One woman told me, "It was difficult to…talk to people who hadn't had this. They could probably sympathize but they couldn't empathize." Another survivor described how a recently diagnosed woman came up to her and "just sobbed and sobbed and sobbed, saying 'I don't think I can do this. You're the only person who even has a rough idea of what I'm thinking.'" While a primary goal of the breast cancer movement was to create support systems for diagnosed women, pink ribbon culture appropriated these efforts to use women's solidarity to galvanize the culture. If diagnosed women believe they need support but that only other survivors can provide it, then joining the sisterhood is the only viable option. Yet pink ribbon culture marginalizes those who do not faithfully comply with the rules of survivorship, leaving these women to turn to existing social networks, most likely the family.

Whereas the idea of social support in pink ribbon culture is highly visible, care work in the family is not. David Karp explains that over time, American society has come to see the family unit as the natural center for helping people who cannot function on their own for whatever reason. This is especially true for those who are dealing with unusual circumstances or some kind of life crisis. Families regularly provide care for disabled children, assist teens who are pregnant, help family members who are divorced or separated, take care of the elderly, and care for those who are sick.[2] Many of the responsibilities involved in non-routine care situations are similar to those provided regularly within the household: cooking, cleaning, doing laundry, grocery shopping, providing childcare, and all of those chores involved in household and family maintenance. When someone is diagnosed with a serious chronic illness, daily household routines usually change. How much they change, and for how long, varies based on the context.

Because women often fulfill caregiving roles in their personal and professional lives, caring tends to be thought of in terms of feminine attributes such as nurturing, empathy, selflessness, and service to others—the love behind the labor.[3] When women get sick, the typical care relationship is reversed. Instead of providing care to others, women need care for themselves. Women typically provide the bulk of care work in the family and in society more generally, so ideas about the proper roles for women as nurturers and caregivers can be a strong influence on a woman's capacity get help for herself when she needs it.[4] As diagnosed women sort out the feeling rules of survivorship, they also manage relationships and social interactions both to take care of themselves and to get care.

The following story of a 51-year old breast cancer survivor illustrates the limits of social support for diagnosed women both within pink ribbon culture and within the family. Natalie, who is married and has a teenage daughter, had an intimate awareness of the physical and emotional suffering that can result from breast cancer and treatment. She also knew that, unlike commonly held beliefs about the role of screening and early detection, mammograms were not always successful in detecting breast cancer early, if at all. Natalie's knowledge about the illness stemmed from her personal experiences with her mother's late-stage diagnosis, 5 years of treatment, and eventual death. By the time Natalie's mother had been diagnosed with invasive breast cancer, the cancer had spread to her heart and bones. Prior to the diagnosis, she had been concerned about a thickening in her breast, but diagnostic tests revealed nothing abnormal and her doctor told her not to worry. Natalie lived with and cared for her mother from the time of her diagnosis to her death.

Two years after her mother died, Natalie noticed a thickening in her breast and went to the doctor. Nothing was visible on a mammogram or computed tomography (CT) scan, and the doctor told her it was probably a fatty tumor and she should forget about it. Because Natalie recognized this sequence of events as analogous to her mother's, she demanded a biopsy. Within a few days Natalie was diagnosed with infiltrating lobular carcinoma, the second most common type of invasive breast cancer in the United States. Natalie immediately started to relive her mother's experience. She cried and wondered if she too would die. She said, "Emotionally, I knew what I went through with my mother. I didn't want my daughter or my husband to have to deal with that. So, I stayed strong, didn't ask for help, and kept going on my own. I'm a fighter." Natalie's strength, resolve, and self-proclaimed warrior status resemble the she-ro. The she-ro identifies with pink ribbon survivorship and defines self-reliance in terms of empowered, self-determined living within pink ribbon culture. Within Natalie's life circumstances—which include memories of her mother's experience, traditional gender roles, and strong feelings of maternal responsibility—self-reliance was defined differently: it meant taking care of herself outside of pink culture, without much help from the family unit or from anyone else.

Natalie's self-sufficiency enabled her to minimize disruption to her daily life and relationships, contributing to a shallow support system. She deliberately tried to handle her life with breast cancer on her own to avoid being a burden to others, but it came at a cost. When I asked Natalie who cared for her at home and what they did, here is what she said:

> Nobody really cared for me. I cared for myself...I didn't really ask for anything. I didn't really expect anything either. I was surprised that more people didn't reach out. I mean, somebody could have offered to watch my daughter for the weekend when I was feeling well so that my husband and I could have some much needed time together. But, they didn't. And, it wasn't like we would ask for it. I mean, I didn't need it...but it would have made our lives much better if we'd had it... things like that. Instead, I did everything on my own...I felt I could handle it. I didn't want to be a burden to anyone.

Natalie defines her needs as the minimum resources necessary to maintain basic physical health, which primarily involves following her breast cancer treatment protocols. Beyond this, she does not feel entitled to any kind of social support that would enhance her quality of life. Sure, help with practical needs such as childcare would be welcome, but for Natalie this is warranted only when it meets a basic need. Instead, Natalie suppresses her own needs to focus on providing a good quality of life for her daughter and her husband. Such self-reliance enables Natalie to maintain gender expectations that call for women's sacrifice and family maintenance. A life situation like Natalie's is not conducive to she-roic survivorship.

The breast cancer movement was successful in bringing breast cancer into the public spotlight and empowering millions of women to claim their status as survivors, but it has not been successful in eliminating the stigma associated with the disease. She-roic women normalize breast cancer and gain status when they identify with the survivor role and present themselves in ways that restore femininity. The she-ro uses breast cancer as a catalyst for transformation, incorporates breast cancer into her life, embraces pink ribbon survivorship, and openly uses the discourse of pink ribbon culture to give meaning to her illness. Although many women do not follow the she-ro model, normalization has become the socially acceptable response for survivors. Natalie, for example, openly incorporates the fighting optimism of pink ribbon culture inherent to the "you can beat this" attitude. Beyond this, she-roic survivorship does not work with her values, history, or the knowledge about breast cancer she gained from her mother's experience. Natalie does not claim her status as a survivor and incorporate breast cancer and pink ribbon culture into her life. Instead, Natalie suppresses her needs for the sake of others, controls her feelings, and normalizes her self-presentation *not* in the name of the ribbon, but in spite of it.

Natalie's motivation is to keep her life and her relationships just as they were before she was diagnosed, not to transform them. She does her best to stabilize life for those around her, minimize the impact of her illness, and suppress her fears. In a matter-of-fact manner, she said several times during our lengthy conversation, "I didn't ask for anything, and I didn't really get anything." Unlike the she-ro who assertively arranges her life to deal with breast cancer, works through her fears, and sets up a support system, Natalie faces continued stigma and a lack of social support. She describes two interactions with her mother-in-law that reveal how normalization enables stigma and diminishes support. Here is the first:

> [My mother-in-law] didn't want to know about it. She was afraid of it. She did watch my daughter sometimes…but otherwise she would just step back. I think she was afraid. And, it hurt me. I didn't have my own mother to comfort me, and she could have filled in, but she didn't. One time, when I was getting a bald spot in the back of my head, she said, "You better go get a wig." I said, "I don't want a wig! If I'm going to be bald, then I'll just be bald, or wear a scarf or something!"… She had to act like I didn't have it, and seeing me without hair wouldn't allow her to do that. I was very hurt. I still am.

In rejecting her mother-in-law's demands that she get a wig, Natalie tried to resist normalization. She wanted her mother-in-law to confront her breast cancer, not because she wanted to gain status as a survivor but because she simply wanted her mother-in-law to acknowledge the illness. Shortly after the wig conversation, Natalie did start to wear a wig. She and her mother-in-law continued to go about their business as usual, thereby limiting opportunities for Natalie to obtain any kind of social support from her.

Throughout her experience with breast cancer, Natalie faced ambivalence about whether she was entitled to receive support from her family. Even at the onset of her chemotherapy treatment, when she was most distressed about how to manage her full-time secretarial job, take care of her teenage daughter, maintain the household, uphold her marriage, and deal with the side effects of treatment, those in a position to help only occasionally came forward to offer it. This heightened Natalie's feelings of isolation and disappointment as she tried to come to terms with how to deal with breast cancer. Natalie shared another devastating interaction she had with her mother-in-law:

> I was about to go to chemo and [my mother-in-law] was heading off for a vacation. She called to say goodbye. There I was...about to go to chemotherapy. She could have offered to watch my daughter, or do something...but instead she was going on a vacation. I still talk to my husband about it. He says, "My family is just not that way. They don't get all involved in everything." I guess its how [he was] raised. But, I was still hurt.

Natalie's understanding of the situation was individualized, explained in terms of how her husband was raised and how his family operates. Natalie's mother-in-law went about her regular activities, including taking a vacation. This was her way of dealing with Natalie's breast cancer and, according to Natalie's husband, was an expected response.

Throughout her experience with breast cancer Natalie did not want to ask for anything that did not fall into her category of absolute necessity. She handled her responsibilities autonomously and lowered her expectations for support. One might argue that Natalie made it possible for those around her to conclude that she did not need help because she went on with her routine and took care of most things on her own. She said:

> I work part time so that I can be home when my daughter's bus arrives from school. I stopped working for three weeks following my surgery. Then, I was right back at work. I did everything I did before. I just did it slower. And, now I know that I can't necessarily get it all done. Some things just have to slide. If the house doesn't get cleaned, then it doesn't. If the work isn't finished when it's time to go home, then it isn't…

Natalie's husband drove her to chemotherapy treatments and did the laundry. Natalie's mother-in-law occasionally provided childcare. Natalie's sisters cooked a meal after each chemotherapy treatment when nausea left Natalie unable to cook for her family. Natalie's daughter maintained her normal routine. Natalie neither asked for, nor expected, any other kind of help.

Still, her long-held disappointment in family members who did not anticipate her needs and reach out to her more suggests that Natalie did want support. In fact, Natalie told me that she periodically reminded her husband that he had no idea how much she had done on her own to keep going. Natalie recognized that she wanted and needed more help than she received, and she has not yet resolved this incongruity. Ultimately feeling the weight of optimism, she neutralized her disappointment with the words, "I guess I should get over it."

Many of the women I have interviewed handled breast cancer the way Natalie did. They maintained optimism and listened to the advice of those who would say, "Don't worry about it, you'll be okay, you're a fighter." They normalized their illness and used formulas for evaluating how severe their illness was, comparing their situations to others who were "worse off." They read about exemplary survivors in pink ribbon culture who "went through the same thing" and were fine. Diminishing how sick they were or how much help they needed did not lead to she-roic empowerment or personal transformation. It enabled women to decrease the level of support and care they thought they should expect or desire. Natalie relied on herself in part because few people reached out to her. She worked to minimize breast cancer's disruption on the lives of those around her and had few opportunities to access support. For women like Natalie, there is an imbalance of care. She supports others, and few people support her. This can work for a time. Selfless women are practiced in going without. If a woman's experience with breast cancer and treatment is severe, however, there is usually an attempt to achieve some kind of balance. Even Natalie said, "[Breast cancer] was a terrible experience…I lived through it once…But, I don't know that I could live through it again…I'm not sure I could get through it a second time."

THE BALANCING ACT

Breast cancer disrupts taken-for-granted assumptions about women's selfless obligations to others. During diagnosis, treatment, and aftercare, women learn to renegotiate their responsibilities and obligations to focus on their own needs for the sake of their health. Then they relearn it, over and over again. The guilt associated with focusing on oneself for too long or from feeling like one is a nuisance to others manifests in different ways, such as holding out the promise of future reciprocity or seeking others' approval for one's uncharacteristic self-interest. When self-reliance no longer works, there is a need for a new ethic of caring that centers on balancing one's needs with the needs of others, and developing strategies to maintain it. Forty-eight-year-old Amy said it best: "There's a good way to be sick and a bad way to be sick."

The rules of survivorship specify how to feel (Chapter 6) and how to do (take on the role of) survivorship. If a woman cannot take care of herself, doing survivorship means learning how to be sick "in a good way," a moral evaluation grounded in social expectations about gender and the broader cancer culture. In other words, diagnosed women attend to the rules of survivorship alongside demands to maintain their roles and identities as selfless and empathetic nurturers. Working within or outside of breast cancer culture, women strive to establish meaningful ways of dealing with breast cancer that mesh with their values, responsibilities, and family situations. Recalling the stories of Ruby and Barbara, and introducing many new voices, the remainder of this chapter reveals how women regularly engage in a balancing act as they set boundaries on what they do for others, and establish criteria about when to accept and ask for help.

Setting Boundaries

In Chapter 6, the feeling rule of selfishness described how diagnosed women should feel about putting their needs first to deal with breast cancer, and then what they should do about how they feel. For the she-ro, selfishness was a justified, rational, and necessary way to take care of herself. However, gender expectations for women's selflessness encourage feelings of selfishness any time women place their personal needs above the needs of others. When Ruby says, "I've become selfish in the way that I know I need to take care of myself," she exposes the disconnection between the social norms that dictate women's selflessness and the practical necessity of focusing on her needs to deal with breast cancer and treatment.[5] Although pink ribbon culture promotes the idea that breast cancer is a valid justification for self-interest, the women I interviewed needed to develop ways to be constructively selfish, given their personal circumstances, roles, and responsibilities. Perceptions about the severity of their diagnoses provided a frame of reference for determining what their needs and priorities were, with the ultimate goal of preventing pain and suffering. Beyond this, women had to learn and relearn how to put themselves first and curb their obligations to others.

Setting boundaries by saying "no" was a fundamental way to mitigate others' needs, desires, expectations, and demands. It was also one of the most difficult things for women to do. Barbara, whom I introduced in the previous chapter, rejected the she-ro model and was committed to dealing with breast cancer on her own terms. This autonomy and self-determination required negotiation and consistent effort within her social environments. Barbara's social networks relied on her caring and generosity and were not ready for her to become selfish, which was really only a reconsideration of how she spent her free time. For example, after she was diagnosed with breast cancer Barbara tried with much difficulty to extricate herself from a volunteer position. She was a treasurer for a local community organization. After her diagnosis she realized that she would have to give up some things. She thoughtfully and responsibly "tied up loose ends" prior to her surgery, and then she tried to resign. She said:

> After I was diagnosed, I spent about a week working on the
> annual report. I did it in July before my lumpectomy because

I didn't want to burden somebody else with that job. I had been treasurer for the year. I tried to keep up the work after that, but I told them I couldn't do this now, and they'd have to get somebody else.

Initially, Barbara felt responsible for the annual report because she believed it was a difficult job, a "burden" in fact. But after her treatment began Barbara felt she could no longer keep the job. The organization found a temporary replacement, but apparently they assumed she would return to the job as soon as she was feeling better. Barbara reiterated: "I told them to tell whoever took it over that I was not going to take it back, because my priorities have changed and I'm going to want to spend my time differently." Despite Barbara's insistence, members of the organization continued to pressure her, telling her that they "have so few people to work on things" and that they "need" her. The service relationship had been established: the organization needed Barbara, and Barbara's needs would not be taken into account, regardless of her breast cancer diagnosis, her surgery, or her personal wishes to reprioritize her activities.

With its focus on triumphant survivorship, pink ribbon culture homogenizes women's experiences in the public imagination while gender expectations demand that women serve others. Common imagery of breast cancer depicts the she-roic survivor who does it all while triumphantly fighting and beating the disease. Similar to the superwoman ideal in which the modern woman efficiently meets the needs of others in all spheres of her life, the she-ro actively takes control of her experience and does not burden others in the process. Taken together, these social forces suppress the capacity of diagnosed women to make their own meaning of breast cancer and live deliberately. Pink ribbon culture also presents breast cancer as a one-size-fits-all situation in which breast cancer is found early when it is most treatable. Barbara was diagnosed with inflammatory breast cancer, and she knew it was rare (representing 1 to 3 percent of cases in the United States) and aggressive (typically diagnosed at stage 3 or 4). With imagery of pink survivorship saturating the cultural environment, the organization was not likely to have this information unless Barbara shared it.

Still reeling with the news of her diagnosis, Barbara was not ready to discuss the reality of her prognosis and she wasn't sure it was anyone else's business anyway. The organization kept hounding her to keep volunteering. She did not give in to the pressure, but making her refusal stick required repeated conversations with different members of the organization. Again and again Barbara told each person who called her that while she had agreed to the job in the past, she was not going to keep doing it. Even the president of the organization called Barbara at home to encourage her to reconsider.

To this point, Barbara said no in a calm but assertive way. She explained to everyone she talked to that her priorities needed to change. Barbara was unsure about how to say no, but she was firm in her decision to do so. The call from the president was the proverbial last straw. She changed both her tone and the information she revealed:

> The president called me and said, "Is there any chance that you will take the treasurer for next year?" I said, "I hate to say so, but no, I'm not going to take it. It's a hideous job that nobody wants...Why should I take a job that everybody hates when my time is most likely limited?"

Knowing that she had a negative prognosis, Barbara finally revealed to the organization that she had an illness that would potentially shorten her life. In our conversations, Barbara said many times that her "life is going to end a lot sooner than [she] thought it would." Her use of the present tense revealed a sense of urgency, which only exacerbated her feelings of exploitation when the organization would not take no for an answer.

Continuing her discussion of the president's phone call, Barbara continued to explain her refusal. She said, "They can pay somebody to do it if they have to. Why should I be the sucker? Let somebody else be the sucker. I tried to do a good thing. I did my share. I told them to give me a small job, and I'll do it." Barbara believed that her refusal to continue the volunteer work was warranted, that the organization acted inappropriately, and that she had already done enough service. She believed she was entitled to say no, to set a boundary that would enable her to take care of herself in the time she had left. Still, Barbara believed that she needed to justify her decision even to me. After getting the message across to the president, she ended up accommodating the organization by taking a small job. The social pressures that women serve others even when facing a life-threatening illness reverberated throughout my interviews, making it difficult for women to set boundaries that would allow them to put their health first.

Ruby had a similar experience at work after being diagnosed with ductal carcinoma *in situ*. As a per diem nurse, Ruby works on a prescheduled basis or sometimes as needed on a day-to-day basis. She had been accustomed to trading shifts with other nurses if they had scheduling conflicts or got sick. Frequently, she would work on what had been a scheduled day off. After her diagnosis and mastectomy, Ruby was not back to her routine. Having worked for several days in a row, she was scheduled for a day off. When she got a request to replace someone, Ruby declined. She tried to say no in an accommodating way while maintaining her identity as a giving person. In fact, Ruby shared a template she uses for saying no that involves expressing remorse about saying no, and then holding out the possibility of saying yes at some point in the future. If someone asks Ruby to work and she does not want to do so, she says, "Well...I just worked three days in a row. I am sorry I can't help you out this time, but maybe next time I can help you." Expressing regret along with the desire to help others enables Ruby to put her needs first.

Setting boundaries is an ongoing process that must be learned. The difficulty women had setting boundaries rests upon deeply embedded norms about women's nurturance, empathy, and selflessness. Women were better able to set boundaries and make them stick if they had some kind of a sounding board (from family, friends, neighbors, coworkers, or support group members) to validate their choices, even if they seemed like relatively minor choices. Sharon, age 70, was diagnosed with invasive breast cancer 1 year before her retirement. During her year of treatment, she did not want to be photographed. Unlike the numerous depictions of smiling survivors in pink head scarves, Sharon did not want to remember this period of her life, nor did she want others to remember it. She felt strongly about her decision, but she was uneasy about how to enforce it. She asked her son how she could keep others from taking her picture, especially during important occasions. He said simply, "Don't let anybody take your picture if you don't want them to." Sharon's son reassured her that it was her right to determine whether or not to be photographed, which strengthened her resolve to set this boundary. He also ran interference at family events so Sharon would not have to defend her choice to others.

Accepting Help

Sixty-year-old Belinda became a widow just a few weeks prior to her breast cancer diagnosis. She had two grown children, and before her husband died they owned two small equestrian-related businesses in a rural community. Having worked dawn to dusk for most of her life, Belinda was independent, resilient, and experienced in selflessness. In many ways, she believed that these qualities enabled her to survive breast cancer. She said,

"Women, I think, are far stronger emotionally than people give us credit for." She gave an example:

> If you're a mother and you're at home and one of the children is sick…No matter how bad you feel, you're taking care of that child. You're up in the middle of the night, giving them juice and what have you…[that] doesn't change just because you got breast cancer.

For Belinda, her business was now her child, and her deceased husband could no longer play a role. She said, "I knew that I had a business to run. I knew that I had one day a week that I couldn't work at it [because I had to go for treatment], but the rest of the time I worked." Belinda's selflessness and work ethic had merged such that she did not allow herself too much time to focus on her sadness or her fears. She said:

> There were times, *I won't deny it*, there were times eight, nine, ten o'clock at night I'd sit here and cry. But sometimes it's better to get that out of your system than to keep it bottled up…I had a friend who once said, "Yup, have a pity party for yourself and put a time limit on it. At two o'clock the pity party is over. Get back to work." (emphasis added)

Belinda acknowledges her emotions and sees the benefit of letting them out. Yet her narrative reflects the optimism rule at work, revealing ambivalence about whether a woman with cancer should admit to feeling sad or sorry for herself. She quickly shifts the discussion to the problem-solving mode she uses to snap herself out of it—"get back to work." This was Belinda's favorite phrase, and she referred to it several times throughout our conversation. It was important for Belinda that she did not present herself as a helpless or fragile woman.

Like many women, Belinda was experienced in actively suppressing her needs for the needs of her children, her business, her housework, her husband, and her family. After being diagnosed with breast cancer, she started to think about what she needed and wanted for herself. This is the part of Belinda's story that resembles she-roic transformation.

> I do things now that I never would have done: (1) if my husband were living and (2) if I hadn't had breast cancer. I was never one to go out and socialize, yet I became the Reach to Recovery lady to go out and talk to other women. Then, I became the Reach to Recovery *trainer* [her emphasis] where I trained other women. I found that to be very fulfilling... Never would I have done that before. It would have been work, work, work.

The formal support systems in place for diagnosed women, such as the Reach to Recovery program sponsored by the American Cancer Society, give women opportunities to learn coping strategies as well as socialize with other survivors. From a sociological perspective, socializing is a primary means of socialization—a way to teach newcomers the rules of engagement within particular social environments. As discussed in previous chapters, cancer culture teaches the diagnosed how to be model survivors. Individuals must then discern for themselves whether the standard modes of survivorship work for them.

For Belinda, socializing was something new, and she liked it. Having recently become a widow, she was not used to living alone. These new social interactions helped her to fill a void.

Belinda developed new friendships, learned about others' experiences, and began to think about her own needs and wants for the first time in her life. This even whittled away at Belinda's habitual self-reliance, as she began to think about what it meant to accept help from others. She attended support group meetings and learned specific techniques. She said, "One of the things we talked about was the fact that women should accept help from family and friends. Somebody wants to bring you a casserole for supper, say yes. Even if you're not hungry for it that night, put it in your refrigerator and heat it up the next day."

The techniques were useful, but Belinda's selfless disposition made it difficult for her to be on the receiving end of caring relationships, and she knew this. She said, "It's difficult to accept help…you do learn to accept the help…isn't that what our life is all about? Do unto others as you would have others do unto you? Still, it's hard to accept." The strong cultural connection between femininity and nurturance creates an ethic of caring that constructs women as caregivers, not the other way around. Women had to learn how to be care-receivers, not in the sense of getting medical care but in their personal lives. The support group gave Belinda reinforcement that it was okay to accept help, but martyrdom was a hard habit to break. Belinda justified accepting help because it reinforced her Christian belief in the Golden Rule. Similarly, most women felt they needed to justify *when* and *if* another's acts of kindness were warranted.

Elaine also admitted that "the whole receiving thing is hard," but she learned to accept help if she believed that the giver enjoyed the giving. She told me a funny story about how a friend tricked an acquaintance of theirs into giving her a gift:

> One day we were talking [about my husband] and she said, "What do you mean your husband's not giving you a massage?" I said, "He's never given me a massage, ever." She said, "Well, that's just horrible." We were walking up the street… we ran into this guy we know…she says, "Rick…Do you give [your wife] massages?" And he goes, "Well yeah…" She says, "Oh that's great. How about you give Elaine a massage? She never gets a massage and she needs one…" He said, "Thank you. I've been wanting to do something for Elaine and I just didn't have a clue. Thank you. I will be glad to give you a massage. I'm coming over to your house. Tell me what day…" He came over…And, he gave me the most incredible massage, even worked on my bald head.

While it took an assertive friend and an odd twist of fate for Rick to give Elaine his gift, Elaine told me later that she practiced daily mantras to learn to accept help from others. She recounted one of her chants: "People are giving you a gift. Do you realize how wonderful it feels when you give a gift to someone? That's how wonderfully they are feeling right now." Elaine's mantra echoes the Golden Rule Natalie believes in. Both of these techniques are strategic explanations for what appears to them to be an imbalance of care. Accepting help, care, support, or gifts from others is appropriate for women only when it is a way to "do unto others."

The she-ro of pink ribbon culture emphasizes strength, courage, and self-interest as women organize their lives around breast cancer and galvanize an army of supporters to win the fight. For many women, however, the realities of their lives do not reflect this vision. Despite the fact that women do learn to set boundaries and to accept help, there are limitations to their success based on social expectations about gender and the nature of caring as something women do for others. Whether from spouses, children, siblings, neighbors, coworkers, or friends, most of the women I interviewed did not have a high tolerance for accepting help. Being sick "in a good way" required a code of conduct that included making others feel comfortable and maintaining good relations. Here's how Amy explained it:

> I don't always look after myself first. I mean, I make sure I have everything I need, [and do what I] need to do, but I always look after other people too…I think if you ask people too much to help you, you become a nuisance when you're sick.

Being independent, placing limitations on one's service, and accepting help under appropriate conditions are processes that do not directly impose upon others. On the contrary, asking for help is an assertive way to encourage others to do what you want.

Asking for Help

When caring for others, it is socially acceptable for women to act assertively on others' behalf. Being an agent for oneself runs counter to women's socially expected roles as caregivers. Ruby stressed this point. After her mastectomy, Ruby's daughter stayed at her house for 2 weeks to help out. Ruby was not able to move very well. She had two drainage tubes stitched to her body beneath her left arm that were designed to collect fluid from the wound. She could not raise her arm, and the drainage bags needed to be emptied every day. It became clear to Ruby's daughter that Ruby was struggling to do things for herself, such as reaching to get a newspaper or trying to get a glass of water. Finally, Ruby's daughter said, "Mom, what do you want? It's okay to ask." Ruby had not realized that she was avoiding asking for help. After her daughter brought it to her attention, Ruby realized, "When it's your time to get help *for yourself*, it's very difficult to ask for it." This difficulty was visible in the many negotiations, frustrations, tensions, and even resentments women discussed throughout their narratives.

Accepting help and asking for it both negate the selflessness associated with femininity. If women are socialized to focus on the needs of others, it is not surprising that they may have little experience defining and articulating their needs. Fifty-seven-year-old Cheryl had been diagnosed with breast cancer 10 years prior to our interview, but her experience remained vivid. In addition to side effects from her treatment, she recounted a lack of support from family. She remarked, "Nobody…my aunts, my cousins…nobody would call and say, 'Can we do anything for you?'…It's kind of hard to ask for help, and when you ask for help and you don't get it…it makes you kind of bitter." Whereas some women are self-reliant because they want to minimize disruption for those around them, bitterness can set in when those close to them fail to notice that they need help. These women are not in a position to think about whether or not help is warranted. Help is not forthcoming. Asking for help and being rejected exacerbates women's feelings that they are not entitled to care, increases isolation, and adds to the stress of having breast cancer.

Cheryl did not receive enough support from her husband either. Cheryl was especially upset about his inability to advocate for her with her doctors. The following excerpt illustrates Cheryl's incapacity to fully define and convey her needs to her husband, and how well-meaning people may not know what diagnosed women need or how to provide it. Such cross-communication can lead to the resentment and frustration Cheryl describes here:

> [My husband] will go to the doctor with me, not every doctor, but he does go to the oncologist with me. He'll go. He's there, but he doesn't really like to ask questions or anything…he's just there. Sometimes I get annoyed because it gets tiring to advocate for yourself all the time. You just want somebody

else to do it for awhile, and I don't get that from him. But, he's not a computer person, so I can't expect him to go on the computer and try to research things. But sometimes I'm just wondering, can't you do something?

Cheryl would like her husband to advocate on her behalf, but she does not ask him to do this. Instead she thinks about how this type of support would be beneficial and attempts to justify her husband's inability to provide it. Despite Cheryl's desire to accept the justification that her husband does not have the capacity to be an advocate, because he is not a "computer person" who can adequately research relevant information, she remains disappointed with the reality that her husband is not providing the kind of support she needs. In some respects, Cheryl suggests that his effort is insufficient as well. It is not that he cannot ask questions; he just doesn't like to ask questions. Her husband's preferences supersede her needs for support.

Generally speaking, women who perceived their diagnosis to be severe were more likely than other women to feel justified in accepting and/or asking for help. Alice, for example, saw her breast cancer diagnosis to be a major life-threatening situation. This allowed her to maintain a commitment to herself and change her expectations of others, including her husband. She said:

I have a husband who looks at me in a very different light now. I never used to think of myself. Growing up with the nuns, get married, sacrificing all these things...now I say, "No, I'm not cooking dinner tonight, you're going to take me out." And, he says, "Okay."

In contrast, Donna perceived her illness to be less severe. She had been widowed for several years and was accustomed to taking care of her grown son, who still lived at home. After her diagnosis, Donna was very grateful that her sister-in-law gave her *no choice* but to live with her family during her treatment. She said:

> I stayed with [my brother and his wife] through my first chemo...then...came home...until I started getting sicker... They didn't...want me to come home at all, but my son [was] by himself. You know how [men] take care of a house...For [my sister-in-law] to take me into her home...was unbelievable. They didn't give me a choice...I was very lucky...I didn't want to have [a stranger] coming into my home and taking care of me.

Aligned with traditional gender expectations, Donna believed that women in families are the appropriate caregivers. She also believed that care requires a uniquely feminine trait, empathy. She did not want her son who was still living at home to take care of her or the household. She was able to have her needs met without having to ask for it, because her sister-in-law (not her brother) insisted. Reinforcing a general lack of entitlement to care, Donna demonstrates remorse. She emphasizes that her sister-in-law's generosity and care are a stroke of fortune rather than a deserved act of family care. What's more, Donna's sister-in-law anticipated her needs. Donna did not have to take care of herself or assertively ask for help.

Even though many women were particular about from whom they were willing to accept help, many were like Donna. They simply had an easier time accepting help when others noticed a need and took action without requiring them to ask. When Amy's husband was proactive in helping with the housework, she was extremely thankful:

> My husband…if something needs [to be] done, he'll go do it…[The house] is a lot of work and I can't keep up to it right now because I've been sick too much. I just got operated on last week and I've been operated on like three times in the last two months…so my husband has been helping me…You don't have to worry about, "Oh, [the dishes] are sitting over there, and they need to be done." He still does that for me…if I have a bad day on dialysis he'll get up and get dinner. He's…a very, a wonderful husband…But…most of the time, I try to be as independent as I can.

In Amy's case, it was her husband who provided the help, but the gendered processes remain: women in families are the appropriate caregivers; caring requires empathy; women ought to be selfless. Amy explains that she can't keep up the house *right now* because she's been *sick too much*. Clearly, the house is Amy's domain, and there is some level of sickness through which she can continue to maintain it. Doing so is part of Amy's self-concept, and she derives fulfillment from this. For Amy, allowing her husband to do this work undermines her sense of self while enhancing her husband's status. It is only when she has a *bad* day on dialysis that her husband has to make dinner. When he does this, he gains the credit of being a *very...wonderful husband* in part because care work is not something men are supposed to do.

Alice described this perspective succinctly. She said, "I'd never really been sick in my life. I went to the hospital to have babies and that was it. All of a sudden, I'm sick and my husband is the one taking care of me! I didn't like the idea of a husband being a caretaker." Alice also believed that care work is women's work. It would have been an assault to her husband's masculinity if he were to take on a caregiving role, and it would have been an assault to her femininity if she had allowed him to do so. For many women, putting the needs of others second to deal with breast cancer involves a shift in perspective, one that can potentially change the essence of their relationships. To protect important relationships from the burden of caring, many women prefer to rely on themselves and their own resources instead.

BALANCING THE SISTERHOOD

Determining an appropriate level of reliance on others and the conditions under which it is warranted or requested involves constant consideration and evaluation. Whether from women or men, many of the women I interviewed did not feel deserving *enough* of assistance to make demands without attenuating them or seeking to restore balance in other ways. Even though women had strategic explanations for what they perceived to be an imbalance of care when people helped them, they still felt guilty about it and frequently tried to reciprocate. Regardless of marital status, presence of children, career, age, or education, it was easier to accept help than to ask for it. Many women felt relief when family members or friends anticipated their needs and then acted to meet them. By relying on others to initiate, women were better able to obtain support while maintaining an essence of feminine selflessness.

Gender expectations are strong. As discussed in Chapter 3, pink ribbon culture draws on the gender system to incorporate pink femininity into its symbols, messages, and stories. Essentially feminizing breast cancer beyond the simple acknowledgement that the majority of breast cancers occur in women, the culture integrates norms of feminine selflessness alongside models of triumphant survivorship, thereby encouraging solidarity among survivors, voluntarism, and commitment to the sisterhood. At a time when women try to strike a balance in their caregiving relationships, pink ribbon culture encourages survivors to return to selflessness by giving back to the broader community of survivors.[6]

The phrase "giving back" was spoken repeatedly when I asked women why, for example, they attended support group meetings, participated in breast cancer advocacy, walked in a 5-kilometer "Race for the Cure," offered guidance to women who were newly diagnosed with breast cancer, or were participating in my research study. I was struck by this phrase because "giving back" suggests that first something was given to them, and second that they were returning it to the person(s) who gave it. What exactly had they received, what were they giving back, and to whom? The answers to these questions reveal that women's engagement in formal and informal support to other breast cancer survivors stems from an attempt to gain understanding, as well as to balance self-interest.

Women "give back" to a community of women with breast cancer to build ties with the only people who, they believe, can truly understand their experience, women who have "been through it." This level of understanding was not present within women's other relationships, and women regularly distinguished between those who could "sympathize" but not "empathize." In the search for empathy, women sought understanding from other women, thereby reinforcing the gendered dimension of social interaction in everyday relationships as well as within the context of breast cancer itself. Relationships among breast cancer survivors formed in varied places, from a formal setting like a support group or treatment facility to a serendipitous meeting at work or as women traversed the medical landscape searching for information about diagnosis and treatment. These relationships enabled women with breast cancer to access informational, instrumental, and emotional support that was not readily available to them in other settings. Breast cancer advocacy made such support and interactions possible. However, pink ribbon culture makes use of survivor relationships to keep breast cancer in the public eye, fortify the culture, raise funds, and maintain the status of breast cancer as a women's health epidemic.

Pink ribbon culture is not unlike other types of voluntarism that make the most of civic responsibility and goodwill. In the context of breast cancer advocacy, the gender system, the branding of the illness, the cancer industry, and women's limited sense of entitlement to care, however, the culture's use of women's voluntarism for the cause can be exploitive. Fifty-one-year-old Melinda was committed to giving back by sharing her story as an African American breast cancer survivor. She wanted to encourage African American women to take breast cancer seriously. In addition to having higher mortality rates at every age, African American women are more likely to be diagnosed at advanced stages, and they have lower 5-year survival rates. These women are less likely to have health insurance, good medical care, and access to diagnostic procedures and health education. Melinda said, "One of the problems…is…it's hard to get [the African American community] to deal with any type of health-related programs." Melinda's statement echoes the concerns of the Sisters Network, a national African American breast cancer survivorship organization whose national campaign "Stop the Silence" focuses on a history within the African American community of not discussing cancer and other life-threatening health concerns.[7]

Melinda was committed to increasing awareness among African American women. After awhile, however, her voluntarism started to impede her efforts to find balance in her life and take care of herself. Melinda emphasized this point when she began to recount all of the speaking engagements, interviews, and volunteer work she had been doing during the 2 years prior to our interview:

> [First, I was] a speaker at the "Making Strides" breakfast and there must have been about 500 people…That September, [a local newspaper] (through American Cancer Society) wanted to do an article on it. Then Channel Six did a story because I…volunteered for the Look Good, Feel Better program. Then [another local newspaper] was doing a story on when a coworker gets cancer…It was good to be able to share with people…but…after a while I said, "This is not okay. All of a sudden I'm just so busy again."

Melinda felt personally responsible for sharing her story because she believed that in the African American community "a lot of people are in denial." She did outreach at work and at her church, but Melinda believed that she "got good press" because breast cancer organizations (and media outlets) are trying to increase diversity.

The public spotlight was added pressure. Melinda had been diagnosed with stage 3 inflammatory breast cancer. She had been unable to work for 14 months due to treatment and complications and had a difficult transition returning to work due to fatigue. Then she kept getting calls to speak and participate in breast cancer activities. She said, "I did not want to be the poster woman for breast cancer." Melinda asked herself: "Is this going to be my primary focus to go around and do this, or am I just going to have this be a part of my life…I decided that I just want it to be a part, not my primary focus." In addition to feeling responsible to her community, Melinda also felt responsible for finding balance. She said, "*I allowed myself*…I took the focus off of me and I began to focus on what I could do with other people and helping other people…it's been a struggle" (emphasis added). The sisterhood assumes no responsibility for exploiting Melinda's goodwill; she had to bear the burden of setting boundaries on the sisterhood's intrusion. Such negotiations are a regular part of the survivor experience, especially for women who are committed to broader communities.

FINAL THOUGHTS

The disruptions that breast cancer diagnosis and treatment cause initiate opportunities for women to make changes in their lives and identities. To manage, many women establish and guard a new sense of self. Yet gendered cultural expectations place limitations on women's capacity to maintain a focus on themselves for very long, even when women believe that breast cancer justifies it. Social factors such as gender, care work, and the culture surrounding breast cancer influence survivors' motivations and capacity to get support. This forces women with breast cancer to engage in a balancing act that involves balancing one's

needs with the needs of others in order to be *sick in a good way.*
The balancing act involves setting boundaries and making distinctions between accepting help and asking for it. Such explanations and justifications can be understood only within a gendered situational context that takes into account the importance of balanced reciprocity for women.

While this chapter highlights the role of gender and the difficulties women face when dealing with breast cancer, most of the women presented here negotiated support in the context of heterosexual families, while taking into account the expectations of husbands and children. Outside of the family, women's social networks also reinforce these expectations. Pink ribbon culture creates a set of scripts that position women within a cultural framework that valorizes women's selflessness to the sisterhood while simultaneously engaging a consumerist logic that necessarily focuses on individual choice. As discussed in Chapter 4, this choice involves purchasing practices and a pink lifestyle that does not necessarily empower women to focus on the needs of their everyday lives. The balancing act is a process of re-socialization and a problem-focused strategy that, if successful, is capable of increasing women's sense of control in coping with the uncertainty of illness and increasing their capacity to find adequate support. It requires women to relinquish (to some extent) dominant scripts that construct women's identities in terms of nurturance, including cultural demands to give back to other breast cancer survivors.

NOTES

1. B. Ehrenreich, "Welcome to Cancerland: A Mammogram Leads to a Cult of Pink Kitsch," *Harper's Magazine* (Nov. 2001): 43-53; S. King, *Pink Ribbons Inc.: Breast Cancer and the Politics of Philanthropy* (Minneapolis: University of Minnesota Press, 2006).

2. Marilyn A. McCubbin, "Family Stress, Resources, and Family Types: Chronic Illness in Children," *Family Relations* 37, no. 2 (1988): 203-10; Deborah Paterniti & Kathy Charmaz, *Health, Illness, and Healing: Society, Social Context, and Self* (Los Angeles: Roxbury, 1999); P. Reynolds, S. Hurley, M. Torres, J. Jackson, P. Boyd, & V. W. Chen, "Use of Coping Strategies and Breast Cancer Survival: Results from the Black/White Cancer Survival Study," *American Journal of Epidemiology* 15, no. 2 (2000): 940-4; D. Karp, *The Burden of Sympathy: How Families Cope with Mental Illness* (New York and Oxford: Oxford University Press, 2001); Eleanor Palo Stoller & S. J. Cutler, "The Impact of Gender on Configurations of Care among Married Elderly Couples," *Research on Aging* 14 (1992): 313-30.

3. E. K. Abel & M. K. Nelson, *Circles of Care: Work and Identity in Women's Lives* (Chicago: University of Chicago Press, 1990); F. Cancian & S. Oliker, *Caring and Gender* (Thousand Oaks, CA: Pine Forge Press, 2000); A. Crittenden, *The Price of Motherhood: Why the Most Important Job in the World is Still the Least Valued* (New York: Henry Holt, 2001); H. Graham, "Caring: A Labour of Love," in *A Labour of Love: Women, Work and Caring*, ed. J. Finch & D. Groves (London: Routledge and Keegan Paul, 1983); J. Tronto & B. Fisher, "Towards a Feminist Theory of Caring," in *Circles of Care: Work and Identity in Women's Lives*, ed. E. Abel & M. Nelson (Englewood Cliffs, NJ: Prentice-Hall, 1990).

4. G. A. Sulik, "When Women Need Care: How Breast Cancer 'Survivors' Cope with Being Care-Receivers." Ph.D. dissertation, University at Albany, State University of New York, 2005.

5. G. A. Sulik, "On the Receiving End: Women, Caring, and Breast Cancer," *Qualitative Sociology* 30, no. 3 (2007): 297-314.

6. *Ibid.*, 308-10.

7. Sisters Network, Inc. 2004-2009. http://www.sistersnetworkinc. org/about.asp#news

EIGHT

SHADES OF PINK

In the early 1990s, it seemed as though society was ready to confront breast cancer. Breast cancer activism was starting to gain momentum in extending public outreach, increasing research funding, and gaining a seat at the public policy table. In August 1993, the *New York Times Magazine* published a story about the achievements of the breast cancer movement with the title, "You Can't Look Away Anymore." The caption referred both to the success of the movement in agitating for change, and to the photograph on the cover. "Beauty Out of Damage" is a graphic self-portrait in which the artist and activist, Matuschka, bared her mastectomy scar. Unlike typical images of breast cancer survivors, the explicit nature of the photograph sparked significant controversy about how breast cancer should be presented to the public. Matuschka, who was diagnosed with breast cancer in 1991 and learned later that her mastectomy was unnecessary, focused on increasing awareness about the prevalence of the disease. Frequently unveiling work that revealed her post-mastectomy body, she was devoted to issues of body image for women, and especially for women who had had mastectomies. With a circulation of 1.8 million, the *Times Magazine* article with its shocking cover called out to the public to pay attention.

Matuschka's now-infamous photograph has appeared in hundreds of international publications, books, television shows, and documentaries. Some of the commentary about the photograph accused her of exploitation, but Matuschka told interviewers that her photographs were not created with the expectation of financial gain. So, why did she do it? The artist says why in a response in *Glamour Magazine* later that year:

> I have always adhered to the philosophy that one should speak and show the truth, because knowledge leads to free will, to choice. If we keep quiet about what cancer does to women's bodies, if we refuse to accept women's bodies in whatever condition they are in, we are doing a disservice to womankind.[1]

Since its cover debut, "Beauty Out of Damage" received 12 awards, including a Pulitzer Prize nomination. The silence that once surrounded breast cancer had been broken.

Fifteen years after the *Times Magazine* confronted the "anguished politics" of breast cancer, representations of breast cancer are everywhere. Pink ribbons and talk of breast cancer awareness in everyday social spaces must mean that, unlike the dark and quiet past, we now have an exhaustive number of ways to show and speak the truth about breast cancer. Regrettably, women and their support networks are now hidden beneath a barrage of pink ribbons and silenced in a cacophony of pink talk. The accepted discourse of pink ribbon culture—solidly lodged in war metaphor, triumphant survivorship, pink consumption, and narratives of quest and transcendence—limits the words, plotlines, and imagery available to communicate women's varied experiences of breast cancer and ways of coping.

THE LIMITING NATURE OF WORDS

After Kristen Garrison's mother died of cancer, she wrote about the difficulty she had writing her mother's obituary. In a scholarly article about breast cancer rhetoric,[2] she wrote:

> Describing her life was easy enough. Describing who survived her straightforward. But I had no words to describe her death, and I stumbled over, resisted, what dad, my sister, and my aunts finally advised: she lost a four-year battle with cancer. I had the most difficulty with the verb.

As a university-level English instructor, Garrison's inability to access words beyond the typical cancer vernacular had nothing to do with her command of the English language. The cancer dictionary has a finite number of words.

Throughout my analyses of breast cancer culture, I have seen and heard the same words over and over again. Courage. Strength. Goodness. Hope. Fight. Survive. Win. These words—along with fear, selfishness, and guilt—cover the pages of this book in a multitude of illustrations and depictions of pink ribbon culture. The war on breast cancer when united with pink femininity leaves few other words from which to choose, and we speak with the words we have. Women write and tell their stories with these words as they continue to fight breast cancer, with the hope that they will win. For many women, the available language is not quite accurate. Beneath their words lies a deeper story that reveals an attempt to communicate differently, to find a more authentic voice.

By far, the most loaded word in the cancer dictionary is *survivor*. Survivor is the label and status of choice in cancer culture, and especially pink ribbon culture. The term refers to anyone who has been diagnosed with and treated for cancer. As discussed in Chapter 2 the role of the survivor emerged in breast cancer advocacy to give voice to diagnosed women, validate their experiences, and give them a role in managing their own health and embodied experiences. In pink ribbon culture, the survivor has become an obligatory status that prioritizes the trauma of suffering, gives the impression that diagnosed women are not dying, and diverts attention from issues related to quality of life while focusing almost exclusively on years survived. These dimensions of survivorship have implications for diagnosed women, and on social understandings of the illness.

Linda is one of the women I interviewed, diagnosed a year earlier, who was not sure whether she should call herself a survivor. She said, "Technically, I'm a breast cancer survivor. But, those who...suffer through chemo, who don't have a guarantee that [breast cancer] isn't going to shorten their life...are the real survivors because it's much harder for them...I don't see myself in that group." The merit of survivorship comes from being a *real* survivor: that is, one who has suffered through the ordeal of breast cancer to come out on the other side, not necessarily unscathed but better off for having had the experience. The image of the triumphant survivor sets the bar of suffering high, making the glory of triumph that much sweeter and deserving of others' admiration. Rather than validating the full range of experience, the survivor model constructs a misery quotient. Did I suffer enough to be called a survivor? Did others suffer more than me? Am I worthy of the sisterhood? In addition to influencing women's capacity to get social support (Chapter 7), such measures invalidate the whole of women's experiences.

The exclusivity of the term *survivor* focuses attention squarely upon those who are living, essentially erasing those who are dying from the disease. The oft-quoted survival rate is the proportion of people diagnosed with a disease who live for a specific period of time. At 5 years, approximately 88 percent of all women diagnosed with invasive breast cancer are alive, meaning 12 percent have died. At 10 years, approximately 77 percent of all women diagnosed with invasive breast cancer are alive, meaning that 23 percent have died. At 20 years, almost half (53 percent) of women diagnosed with invasive breast cancer are alive, meaning that nearly half of them have died. As diagnostic tools detect some types of breast cancer earlier, the 5-year survival rate for that cancer appears to increase, regardless of whether patients actually live longer (called lead-time bias). The incidence rate also increases because more cancers are diagnosed at the sub-clinical (producing no symptoms) stage. This is not simply a matter of looking at the breast cancer glass as half-full (some survived) or half-empty (some died). The term *survivor* is a misnomer, as one woman remarked: "Have I survived? I won't know unless I die of something besides breast cancer. The term is overused."

The term *survivor* not only focuses on those who are living but also on the number of years they have survived. This dimension of survivorship directs attention to life expectancy rather than quality of life. Knowing that someone who was diagnosed with breast cancer is still living many years after the diagnosis can be inspiring to the newly diagnosed, lessening the deeply rooted historical stigma that breast cancer is a death sentence. However, counting the years a person remains alive does not consider the state of her life during those years. Barbara explained a difficult and depressing existence during her chemotherapy treatment. She said, "There was one week when…I was really ready to end it all, when I hadn't slept at all, my legs were rubber, I held onto the walls to walk. I felt so awful. It was the last day of chemo, which is usually the worst….You don't feel great most of the time."

Barbara's suffering would rank her as a deserving survivor, but she did not want to *survive*. She wanted to *live*.

The term *survivor* is commonplace. Most of the women I have met over the years continue to use the term *survivor* to refer to themselves and other diagnosed women. Yet, some women have intentionally tried to recontextualize the meaning of survivorship by using other terms. A monologue-style theater production performed in Albany, New York, called "Alive, Alive, Oh!" was based on the personal stories of 10 local cancer survivors who called themselves "alivers." The production focused on raising awareness of cancer care issues and fostering personal expression of people affected by cancer.[3] Like Barbara, they too wanted to acknowledge a fuller range of experiences and quality-of-life issues than the term *survivor* could accommodate. Similarly, some women call themselves "thrivers" to call attention to their capacity to live valued lives despite their circumstances. These "survivors," "alivers," and "thrivers" develop alternative ways of speaking about breast cancer, and narrating their illness, that more accurately reflect how they get on with their lives.

NARRATING ONE'S ILLNESS

More than simply stories of suffering, *illness narratives* tell the story of an illness and its effects on a person's life. These can be spoken in everyday conversation, written in biographical or auto-biographical accounts, or conveyed through art, music, poetry, prose, or other forms of communication. In *The Wounded Storyteller*, Arthur Frank explains that ill people have to learn to think differently because illness causes them to lose the map that previously guided their lives.[4] The personal stories people tell (and write) about their illnesses help them to construct a new map. In this process, illness narratives assign a function to the illness. Told through a wounded body, illness narratives position the ill person as a witness to his or her own suffering, helping ill people to establish a sense of coherence to their lives. In a 2000 interview for the *Antioch Review*, award-winning American poet and breast cancer survivor Lucille Clifton revealed the redemptive power of illness narratives in her comments about why she writes:[5]

> I think that writing is a way of continuing to hope. When things sometimes feel as if they're not going to get any better, writing offers a way of trying to connect with something beyond that obvious feeling...there is hope in connecting, and so perhaps for me it is a way of remembering I am not alone. And the writing may be sending tentacles out to see if there is a response to that.

As Clifton's remarks suggest, illness narratives affirm ill persons' understandings of their experiences as they read their writing, hear themselves telling their stories, experience the sharing, and absorb others' reactions to what is shared. In these ways, illness narratives symbolically repair the disruption an illness has caused in a person's life.

According to Frank, illness narratives take different forms (restitution, chaos, or quest), each of which chart the story of an illness in a person's life. *Restitution* narratives focus on cure and returning to a previous state of health. This is the narrative that usually surfaces during an acute type of illness, such as the flu, a broken bone, or even the successful surgical removal of a cancerous tumor. The ill person believes that the illness is a temporary disruption, and that life will return to normal. *Chaos* narratives express that things are out of control and will never get better. People with debilitating chronic illnesses such as Alzheimer's disease use this narrative to communicate the disorder of their lives. This narrative serves a vital function in articulating the realities of a chaotic situation induced by an illness. If heard and accepted, ill persons can begin to build new lives. Finally, *quest* narratives use the illness to gain personal insight and engage in personal transformation. The ill person can no longer imagine returning to his or her old self, faces tremendous difficulties, learns from the experience, changes as a result of it, and seeks to share the lessons learned. Stories of triumphant cancer survivorship fulfill this narrative.

In addition to the form an illness narrative takes, cultural contexts provide the discursive tools (words, characters, images, settings, plotlines) that are necessary to narrate the story. For the story to be heard and accepted, ill people must follow certain cultural conventions. Pink ribbon culture, in conjunction with the broader cancer culture, helps shape the illness narratives of those diagnosed with breast cancer. Specifically, the personal story of the survivor gained significant public status by the mid-1990s, and breast cancer narratives became a new genre within mass media. The survivor story took the form of restitution and quest narratives, with the language and imagery of the culture supplying the details. Since cancer culture aligns closely with the cancer industry, the language of medical consumption also helps to frame the story.

The plot of the restitution story is simple: diagnosis, treatment, and cure (typically referred to as being "cancer-free"). Within this narrative, a woman may be "sick" for a while, but she will recover and return to her old self. Descriptions of the most commonly used surgical procedures, which focus on retaining or recreating a feminine body image, promote this story. Unlike the dramatic, disfiguring operations of the past (i.e., the Halsted radical mastectomy, which removed the whole breast, all of the lymph nodes up to the collarbone, and the chest muscles), the model procedures used since the late 1980s have focused on breast conservation. The biopsies frequently used in diagnostic processes (e.g., fine-needle and core biopsies) avoid scarring incisions. The preferred method of treatment for many women with small tumors (under 4 cm) is a lumpectomy (i.e., partial mastectomy), in which the tumor is removed along with some of the surrounding normal tissue and is followed by breast irradiation. For women who have mastectomies, immediate breast reconstruction, using either an implant or tissue from elsewhere in the body, has become more routine, especially for younger women. The breast cancer treatment of today aims to avoid too much breast disfigurement: restore the feminine body ideal, and restore the feminine self.

In some cases, women cannot return to their old self. Surgeries may not turn out as intended; treatment may have too many side effects; recurrences happen; or the cancer is too aggressive to be kept at bay in the first place. The restitution narrative does not work, and the quest narrative takes over. The quest story begins with some kind of call, in which symptoms, diagnoses, or prognoses set a new journey in motion. Initially, most people reject the call because they are confounded with what they think they know about their illness (e.g., "But my breast cancer was found early…they got it all…I had chemo…I did everything right… I was cancer-free for 8 years."). At some point the circumstances, symptoms, or suffering make denial no longer possible. People begin to experience bodily harm, life disruption, or existential trauma in a way that cultivates insight and inspires personal transformation. The triumphant survivor emerges, either having "conquered" breast cancer or having returned from the battle compassionately humbled. Either way, she is ready to share what she has learned with others.

The discourse and imagery that serve pink ribbon culture and the cancer industry—namely, those that emphasize the archetypal story of the triumphant survivor—are most widely circulated in mass media and public awareness campaigns. As the protagonist of the quest narrative, the survivor is a courageous, optimistic, and transformed she-ro who celebrates her survival and offers inspiration and hope to other women. Setting the standard for survivorship, she has become the public voice for breast cancer survivors, drowning out alternative ways of thinking about, and dealing with, breast cancer. The ubiquity of her story makes it difficult to change the terms of the public discussion or the ways of coping it promotes. Still, diagnosed women continually try to find their own pathways of survivorship and authentic ways to communicate their experiences, even if it means selectively using the tools of the culture itself.

Realism and Transcendent Subversion

The value of candid self-expression about one's experience with breast cancer was made public with Matuschka's shocking self-portrait. In this spirit, more than 70 breast cancer survivors contributed to a unique collection art, fiction, poetry, and prose called Art.Rage.Us., an ongoing, traveling exhibit that was published in book form in 1998.[6] The Literature, Arts, and Medicine Database describes the collection as an unabashedly political call to arms:[7]

> Many pieces are provocative and challenge our thinking: Matuschka's self portrait with her mastectomy scar exposed on one side, the other covered with half of a sexy black corset; Diane Young's joyful photograph of seven shirtless women (all close friends) and a female child, one of them with a double mastectomy, entitled "One in Eight"; or Francoise and Denny Hultzapple's black and white photograph of their embrace, Denny's face nestled near her bared scar.

Certainly, the collection is different from mainstream portrayals that demand normalized images of beauty, perfection, and optimism.

The provocative title suggests a new way of thinking about breast cancer that moves beyond common pink ribbon imagery. In its appeal to the senses and emotions, *art* is beyond words opening the potential for new and unrestrained communication. *Rage* allows for the expression of furious anger, something out of the ordinary in a culture of optimism (anger is red, not pink). The contributing artists represent a new collectivity of authentic breast cancer survivors, a new *us* that validates the expression of anger and frustration about breast cancer. The collection offers the audience a rare glimpse of realism. At the same time Art.Rage.Us must contend with the dominant culture. The Breast Cancer Fund collaborated with San Francisco-based chapters of American Cancer Society and the Susan G. Komen Breast Cancer Foundation to produce the collection. Given the centrality of their mother organizations within pink ribbon culture, the selection of works for exhibition and publication would have to speak pink ribbon language to some extent to be accepted by this community. Three of the artworks featured on the Art.Rage.Us Web site, along with statements from the artists who created them, reveal the continued influence of pink ribbon culture on resistant, realistic expressions of breast cancer.

First, in "Circus de Vida" (The Crucified Clown) by Diana DeMille, the colored pencil on wood portrays a self-portrait of the artist as a tragic clown and her life as a circus. The image, saturated with the color red, reveals pain and anger. She is the crucified clown: tempered, tormented, wounded, and subdued. Her face paint hides her expression as she makes an obscene gesture: "Elegantly, imperceptibly, you gesture, afraid to say what you really feel."[8] Her bleeding palm signifies injury. The tightrope act in the background portrays her life as a "balancing act" as she tries to balance her own needs with the needs of those who wish to protect her, her multiple responsibilities with a personal desire for healing and self-care. The piece is a candid depiction of the pain and emotional upheaval caused by breast cancer, and the social and cultural expectations that limit personal expression when dealing with it. The artist explains that she initially tried to cope with her "lopsided scar-slashed chest" by refusing to acknowledge it. For 5 years, she refused to look. Revealing this secret through her painting, DeMille comments that creativity became a way to heal. She shares with the reader that "inner healing cannot begin until the first step is taken: expressing one's anger and rage."[9]

Secondly, professional photographer Kit Morris contributed "Radiation Collage," a collection of images showing the effects of radiation treatment on her skin: the boost circle, the tattoos, and the sunburn. In addition to receiving radiation therapy to the entire breast, women often receive an additional "boost" of radiation to the area that surrounds the cancer. Permanent tattoo markings are used to ensure the accurate targeting of the tumor area and to allow the technician to line up the treatment fields more quickly. Most of the time there is a slight reddening and dryness of the skin. Morris captured these effects with her camera. She said, "Color can be very deductive. As part of my healing process, I photographed. Some of the images were beautiful whereas others were shocking."[10] Revealing a multifaceted picture of both the temporary and lasting effects of radiation on the skin, the photograph gives visual representation to a process that most often stays within hospital walls and effects that remain hidden beneath clothing. Morris goes on to share her insight into the experience: "Having cancer is shocking, but surviving it is a beautiful experience that I am thankful for every day."

In both of these pieces, the artists express realities about breast cancer, which often remain hidden. In "Circus de Vida," DeMille presents herself as a foolish clown, unable to balance her responsibilities or find peace within the spectacle that has become her life. She calls attention to the mask that diagnosed women wear to conceal the emotional upheaval and anger they are not allowed to express, indicating that something truthful exists beneath the mask. The mask described here also reflects the feeling rules of pink ribbon culture, and the emotional turmoil these rules can cause for diagnosed women. Morris' "Radiation Collage" also draws attention to truth, as she shows the real effects of cancer treatment on her skin. Her compilation is a means of preserving various moments of her irradiated body, just as it is. Having revealed the real, both artists then share important insights that came out of their experiences. Realism is framed with enlightenment, a key facet of transcendence within the quest narrative.

Further emphasizing the quest narrative, the brightly colored mixed-media painting "Persephone's Return," by Joyce Radke, depicts a mythic story of transcendence in the image of the Greek goddess Persephone. To know the artist, one must know the story. In Greek mythology Persephone is the daughter of Zeus. She represents fertility, harvest, eternal spring, and innocence. The Greek god Hades abducted Persephone into the underworld to make her his queen. She desperately wanted to return to her life on earth, and eating while in the underworld would result in a permanent stay. Persephone knew this, but when Hades offered her a pomegranate she willingly ate seven seeds. Hades softened at Persephone's gesture and decided to let her spend 4 months each year with him in the underworld (winter) and the remaining months on earth (spring, summer, and fall). The arrangement resulted in a positive outcome, as it created the seasons and a new cycle of fertility.

In Radke's painting, Persephone has a red mastectomy scar. Uniting the goddess' tragic story with her own experience of breast cancer, the artist builds a mythic journey of survivorship in which the story of the goddess presides over the artist's lived experience. Radke writes:

> After I was diagnosed...I became fascinated by...Persephone...I imagine that she felt she had a new chance to find her life again, to embrace the light. Like Persephone, I journeyed in the dark realms and used the seeds of creativity to find my way home. By imagining myself as the goddess of eternal spring, I was able to escape from the pain, the grieving,

the dark and barren landscape the doctors painted for me.
I have returned to the light, to living moments as they come
and embracing every second I have.[11]

Imagining herself as the embodiment of Persephone, Radke
enters the story to live the mythology. Abducted not by Hades,
but by cancer and its treatment, Radke acknowledges the pain
of the journey, the desire to escape, the power to transform, and
the victory of return. The actual details of Radke's experience
lie somewhere beneath the mythic plotline and the ultimate les-
son she learns: to embrace life, and live moment to moment.

The Art.Rage.Us collection has the potential to demystify
the experience of breast cancer and reveal aspects of the illness
that are obscured both in normative social interactions and in
mainstream portrayals. In addition to the three highlighted artworks, descriptions of the collection reiterate the survivor's
quest narrative. A review of the collection on Amazon.com says
that the book "illustrate[s] the strength, fear, passion, anger, and
renewal that comes with the breast cancer experience."[12] In this
version of the epic story, the she-ro does not have a smile on her
face, but she does rise above her experience, enlightened by the
difficult journey. With tenacity and fortitude, she uses her creativity (and her anger) to aid in personal transformation. The
review goes on to outline "the range of emotions" available to
diagnosed women: "dignity, courage, anger, terror, grief, humor
and acceptance."[13] Art.Rage.Us both reinforces and extends the
cancer dictionary. Adding dignity and anger to the list is reminiscent of Matuschka's 1993 "Beauty Out of Damage" self-portrait,

which demanded that we speak and show the truth about breast
cancer. Framing these words with transcendence and homage to
women's courage emboldens the survivor's quest, softening the
truths expressed.

Art.Rage.Us reveals the challenge to convey realism about
breast cancer in the midst of strong cultural conventions. Revered
for its stunning imagery and provocative impact, the collection
provides an outlet for expression in an otherwise closed and sanctioned environment. Several books and collections have used a similar approach. *Winged Victory: Altered Images Transcending Breast Cancer* was
first published in 1996 and then revised and expanded in 2009.[14]
Framed with the personal stories of survivors in France and the
United States, the book shows images of women's postsurgical
bodies to challenge readers to re-envision beauty after breast cancer. *Heroines* is a 2006 collection of black-and-white portraits
and poetry that convey the trials and spiritual transformation of
21 Minnesota women who faced breast cancer.[15] *Reconstructing
Aphrodite*, published in 2001, tells the stories of diagnosed women
who successfully underwent the parallel operations of mastectomy
and reconstruction.[16] Fulfilling restitution and quest narratives, the
women portrayed return to wholeness physically and emotionally,
with personal stories that convey courage, confidence, and connection. These books frame the often-hidden realities of breast cancer
within an accepted cancer lexicon and narrative structure, incorporating and recontextualizing aspects of pink ribbon culture.

The pinking of realism has been a successful strategy for pink
ribbon culture to absorb the anger and outrage that surrounds

breast cancer, a success that is not lost on the cancer industry. In partnership with the National Coalition for Cancer Survivorship, the pharmaceutical giant Eli Lilly and Company launched a biennial art competition in 2004 called *Oncology on Canvas: Expressions of a Woman's Cancer Journey*.[17] The first international competition and exhibition, which focused on women's cancers, had more than 400 entries from 23 countries and toured in over 100 cities worldwide. By 2006, Lilly opened the competition to anyone affected by cancer and renamed the program *Oncology on Canvas: Expressions of a Cancer Journey*. With over 2,000 entries from 43 countries, the global competition and exhibition had grown exponentially, reaching millions of people in over 200 cities worldwide. Lilly reduced its program in 2008, limiting the competition to artists in the United States and Puerto Rico only. This change resulted in almost 600 entries, monetary donations to 20 cancer charities that were selected by the competition winners, and a nationwide touring exhibit to hospitals, cancer centers, patient advocacy group meetings, and other venues.

Oncology on Canvas calls upon industry, advocacy, and culture. Lilly claims that the art competition is to "honor the journeys people face when confronted with a cancer diagnosis." Yet, the word "oncology" does not refer to those who are diagnosed with cancer; it refers to the field of medicine that is dedicated to cancer. The banner on the Web page for the art competition is broken into two side-by-side text boxes.[18] The first box is gray and holds the title "Lilly Oncology." The box next to it is red, with the title "Oncology on Canvas." The word *oncology* that unites the two phrases sends a clear message: Lilly Oncology, on Canvas. The competition is an ideal platform for the medical industry, and a forum for Lilly's public relations as a key player in that industry. The media alert template[19] that Lilly provides to healthcare providers and advocacy groups presents the company as a "world leader in cancer research and treatment," and Lilly's logo flourishes amid the competition's promotional materials in bright-red letters to promote the Lilly Canvas.

These intentional advertising strategies fall beneath the radar as Lilly gains legitimacy from a major cancer advocacy organization. In partnership with the National Coalition for Cancer Survivorship (NCCS), which Lilly reveres as "the oldest survivor-led cancer advocacy organization in the U.S.," the company is able to draw on the history of cancer advocacy in the United States, the social credibility of the survivor role, and the cultural repertoires cancer organizations use to achieve their own missions.

Pink ribbon culture and the broader cancer culture in the United States tend to blur, especially with regard to transcendence as the key to survivorship. In turn, painting a picture of transcendence positively colors any public relations activity. Lilly's media template uses transcendence to establish the tone for the *Oncology on Canvas* exhibit:

> Oncology on Canvas…invites people…diagnosed with any type of cancer, as well as their families, friends, caregivers and healthcare providers, to express, through art and narrative, the life-affirming changes that give the cancer journey meaning.

The outrageousness of cancer that Art.Rage.Us illuminated, though tempered with a transcendent message, gives way to a full-blown rush of affirmation and meaning in Lilly's version of personal expression. The effects of cancer and treatment that are not life-affirming—indeed, those that are disruptive, harmful, life-threatening, and possibly the result of the cancer industry's own products and agendas—are left out of the frame. Likewise, death is not an acceptable part of the survivor's journey.

The Picture Outside the Frame

Transcendence is not a bad thing. It can help to give coherent meaning to illness, increase feelings of connectedness, promote self-care, and improve a person's quality of life.[20] In fact, self-transcendence has been seen as a major psychosocial resource that contributes to physical and emotional well-being, and increases one's ability to manage activities of daily living.[21]

In the psychosocial literature, self-transcendence is defined as the "expansion of one's boundaries inwardly in various introspective activities, outwardly through concerns about others and temporally, whereby the perceptions of one's past and future enhance the present."[22] Recalling earlier discussions of illness narratives—which help ill people to bear witness to their suffering, forge connections with others, and establish a sense of coherence to their lives—illness narratives are a mode of self-transcendence.

As individuals try to make sense of their lives in light of a cancer diagnosis, many people find a deeper understanding of life and its meaning and develop ways to adapt.[23] However, transcendence comes in different varieties. Pink ribbon culture values the affirming survivor story, the one that focuses on Persephone's tale of moving out of the darkness and into the light. It is the ending of the story that matters, rather than the realities of the journey itself, with its light and shadows and many shades of gray. In Matthew Sanford's *Waking: A Memoir of Trauma and Transcendence*, the author tells a story of his experience with traumatic spinal cord injury at age 13 and the ongoing trauma associated with his recovery and adjustment. He explains that throughout the process he dealt with conflicting messages about how to come to terms with the fact that he would not walk again, from others' commands that he simply accept it (i.e., get over it), to a form of acceptance that incorporates a new sense of himself as a whole person who does not walk. In his memoir, he acknowledges the whole of his lived experience.

For example, after practicing yoga for 13 years Sanford developed the capacity to feel a sense of presence, or awareness, in the back of his heels. This is not a sensation of the physical body brought on by nerve impulses, but a perception of feeling in his subtle body. He said: "I marvel at the thought...I am not walking, nor do I feel courageous, but I have worked so hard for such a moment. It has taken patience, persistence, and a willingness to feel vulnerable. It has taken a different kind of strength."[24] Sanford's long-term commitment to sense something so slight and ordinary is indeed a different kind of strength. Seldom does talk of survivorship involve perceptions of embodiment that go beyond medical interventions or activities of daily living. Nor does it typically involve words such as *patience* or *vulnerability*. Sanford's illness narrative is not the typical survivor story bounded in restitution or quest. He cannot return to his pre-paralyzed self or his life as a walking person. He does not present himself as an enlightened person who is better off for having endured the intense struggle of a difficult journey.

I share a glimpse of Sanford's memoir to show how deep social norms go. Ideas about survivorship and transcendence cut across different types of traumatic experiences, as does the pressure to tell certain types of illness narratives. Cancer culture does not have sole ownership of the survivor story and its transcendent frame.[25] The product description of Sanford's book reads like many other survivor stories—an inspirational, powerful message about the endurance of the human spirit. Sanford's story is indeed candid, personal, devastating, philosophical, and spiritual. Yet, it is grounded in a *realistic* narrative that acknowledges and articulates the nuance of illness as a dimension of lived experience. It is a story of a person who achieves transcendence by leaving the transcendent frame out of the story. By recontextualizing cultural expectations for courage, strength, and aggressive action, Sanford acknowledges that surviving trauma, any kind of trauma, sets up a cultural repertoire about how to speak about the experience and give it meaning. In taking charge of his own story, he creates a new pathway for survivorship that is self-determined and authentic. At the same time, the story itself goes beyond Sanford's personal experience to illustrate the essence of a particular human condition.

Many breast cancer survivors are like Sanford, not in terms of mobility, mind–body practices, or beliefs necessarily, but in terms of the desire to tell a realistic narrative that reveals something true about the lived experience of breast cancer. Throughout the development of pink ribbon culture, there have always been realistic illness narratives that grounded the person's survivor story within lived experience to articulate sensed perceptions as well as interpretations of those perceptions. Telling an authentic story about an illness that is heavily laden with cultural expectations about femininity, normalcy, and triumphant survivorship requires a new way of thinking and speaking. Falling on the margins of the cultural framework, these kinds of stories can be threatening and hard to hear.

The Terrible Stories[26]

> *I am a post-mastectomy woman who believes our feelings need voice in order to be recognized, respected, and of use.*
> AUDRE LORDE, THE CANCER JOURNALS[27]

Audre Lorde, African American poet, essayist, autobiographer, novelist, and nonfiction writer, was diagnosed with breast cancer in 1978. Six months after her modified radical mastectomy, she began writing journal entries about her experiences with breast cancer. Lorde published an account of her illness in *The Cancer*

Journals in 1980, which included excerpts from her journal entries. Lorde's writing called for cancer survivors to support one another and speak out about American culture's push to render invisible the devastating impacts of breast cancer on women's bodies, lives, and voices. In a similar vein as Rose Kushner's work, which sought to question medical practice and break the silence that still surrounded breast cancer, Lorde's ability to raise issues that help to initiate social change has had a lasting impact on cancer survivorship. *The Cancer Journals*, republished in 1995 and 2006, continues to serve as a prophetic message for numerous cancer survivors and community-based organizations.

In the first chapter of *The Cancer Journals*, "the transformation of silence into language and action," Lorde emphasizes the importance of illness narratives. Putting what she feels into words enables the ill person to reflect on her experience, examine it, put it into a perspective, share it, and make use of it. Lorde argues forcefully that communicating our experiences not only benefits the speaker on a personal level, but also gives voice to realities that will cause harm if left unattended. She writes:

> I was going to die, if not sooner then later, whether or not I had ever spoken myself. My silences had not protected me. Your silence will not protect you…while we wait in silence for that final luxury of fearlessness, the weight of that silence will choke us.[28]

For Lorde, it is the truthful telling of all kinds of stories that matters, not only those accepted in the broader culture.

Her goal is not to construct a singular Truth, such as the story of the triumphant survivor, but to create opportunities for women to seek out and examine a diversity of stories and consider their relevance to their lives. Coping with illness is related to one's sense of what is possible and acceptable. Personal expectations about how to adapt to illness depend in part on the expectations promoted (or suppressed) in the stories of one's culture.

The second and third chapters share some of Lorde's own adaptive truths. From the time of her initial biopsy in 1977 (benign) to her second biopsy in 1978 (metastasized breast cancer) and mastectomy 3 days after diagnosis, Lorde considered the pros and cons of every possible treatment: holistic, conventional, and alternative. She gave vivid accounts of her biopsies, mastectomy, her refusal to wear a prosthesis, and the decision-making involved in determining the wisest method of treatment. She described her fury that no one had told her about the physical pain she would feel after surgery and a nurse who, visibly disgusted with her screams of pain, sedated her. Lorde's vivid recounting of an interaction she had with a volunteer from the American Cancer Society's Reach to Recovery program clarifies the strong disconnection she had with mainstream approaches to breast cancer:[29]

> A kindly woman from Reach [to] Recovery came in to see me, with a very upbeat message and a little prepared packet containing a soft sleep-bra and a wad of lambswool pressed

into a pale pink breast-shaped pad. She was 56 years old, she told me proudly. She was also a woman of admirable energies who clearly would uphold and defend to the death those structures of a society that had allowed her a little niche to shine in. Her message was, you are just as good as you were before because you can look exactly the same. Lambswool now, then a good prosthesis as soon as possible, and nobody'll ever know the difference. But what she said, was '*You'll* never know the difference,' and she lost me right there, because I knew sure as hell *I'd* know the difference…I needed to talk with women who shared at least some of my major concerns and beliefs and visions, who shared at least some of my language…This lady, admirable though she might be, did not.

Lorde's interaction with the Reach to Recovery volunteer captured the essence of her critique. She was concerned that normalizing women's experience through appearance and artificial restoration gave the medical system permission to pathologize, discipline, and profit from women's cancerous bodies. Such critical perspectives were out of place in the hospital and, according to another nurse, some of Lorde's behaviors were "bad for morale."

Lorde emphasized that normalization and "looking on the bright side of things" functioned as a "euphemism…for obscuring certain realities of life, the open consideration of which might prove threatening or dangerous to the status quo."[30] After sharing a letter she had read in a medical magazine in which a doctor said that "no truly happy person ever gets cancer," she stressed the importance of making a distinction between self-affirmation and the superficial guise of happiness. The centrality of cheerfulness as the primary way to survive cancer succeeds in blaming the diagnosed for getting cancer in the first place, limiting women's personal expression to sanctioned cultural scripts that support the cancer system, and giving society at large an opportunity to look away from the realities of modern living that give rise to cancer and illness, such as environmental causes and profit motives within the medical system that preclude any real investment in prevention.

Lorde's second memoir about her breast cancer experience, *A Burst of Light* (1988), continued her critique of both the feel-good messages about breast cancer and the profit motives of the cancer industry. The book chronicled her choice for noninvasive treatment after the cancer had spread to her liver 6 years after the initial diagnosis. Lorde survived breast cancer for 14 years and died from the disease at age 58. Her experience characterizes a different kind of war against breast cancer, in which the warrior did not fight her own body but rather the social systems that controlled the conditions of her illness. Rekindled in Alexis De Veaux's 2004 biography of Audre Lorde, *Warrior Poet*, these and other social concerns illuminate Lorde's ability to use her personal experiences to articulate broader human processes and political controversies.[31] The struggle to speak authentically about breast cancer continues to plague the culture of survivorship three decades after the publication of her first memoir.

> War, cancer, and death are archetypally real. The urge to soften them, to fend off their reality, to metaphorize them, this urge overpowers our ability to speak the truth.
>
> CHRISTINA MIDDLEBROOK, SEEING THE CRAB[32]

Resisting dominant cultural norms to tell a realistic story about one's experience differs from the way women's magazines and other forms of mass media talk about breast cancer. With a focus on triumphant survivorship and the power of positive thinking, few diagnosed women have the opportunity to write about (or speak about) their experiences with breast cancer outside of quest narratives. When they do, they stand out. *Cancer in Two Voices* by Barbara Rosenblum and Sandra Butler; *Grace and Grit* by Kenneth and Treya Killam Wilber; *Diary of a Zen Nun* by Nan Shin; *Ordinary Life* by Kathlyn Conway; and *Seeing the Crab: A Memoir of Dying* by Christina Middlebrook are vivid stories that describe the realities of living and dying with cancer. As with Lorde's memoirs, these writings give readers a new lexis for describing cancer that captures the disruptive aspects of the illness experience that are most often hidden from public view and a form of transcendence or self-acceptance that does not require the ill person to have an epiphany that transforms her suffering into triumphant survivorship.

In a class I taught on the Sociology of Breast Cancer, I gave my students a list of illness memoirs and asked them to review a book of their choice. Among other things, I asked them to examine the perspectives of the author, the plot, any underlying messages (norms or rules) about how one should cope, why they chose the particular book, and whether they liked it. One of the most interesting reports was on Middlebrook's *Seeing the Crab,* written by a Jungian psychoanalyst from San Francisco who was diagnosed with stage 4 metastatic breast cancer. My student chose the book because it dealt with death, something either avoided or uncontested in contemporary social life. She wanted an account that would help her to better understand the dying process, and how a person could live in the face of impending death.

After reading the book, she was disappointed because she still had no answers for herself about the meaning of life and the ways of death. She believed, though, that she would be more empathetic to people with cancer, instead of falling into the "American denial system" that treats people with cancer as though they will be "just fine." Part of my student's frustration with the book was that the plot was atypical.

First, the timeline and tense shifted continuously. Narrating the illness from diagnosis to remission to recurrence, Middlebrook interrupts the story with memories and flashbacks that shift between present and past tense, leaving the reader with an unstable sense of time. Different from the journalistic style of many personal narratives with a clear beginning, middle, and end, *Seeing the Crab* is written in a way that illustrates the narrator's experience of disruption. In a chapter called "Cooked Carrots" Middlebrook writes:

> Months after the bone marrow transplant, when my hair was still radically short and I was still weak, my friend Chauncy took me for a slow walk. I took her arm as we crossed the six-lane intersection at Lombard and Broderick. "Fucking dykes!" a carload of young blond heterosexuals, all female, yelled at us, proclaiming my return to the world of the healthy. I look normal now. No one calls me names…Can I surrender to life as I once surrendered to cancer treatments?…Time has lost its linear qualities. Every day makes a circle. Each season recalls the season before. At Easter 1994 I remember Easter 1993 and 1992. The little bunny vases are filled with forget-me-nots and pansies. We are eating lavender and turquoise hard-boiled eggs again.

Middlebrook's writing conveys the realities of her life, interrupted by the physical, practical, emotional, and symbolic changes that result from her illness. In attempting to make sense of her own story with all of its fits and starts, she gives the reader an opportunity to do the same.

Second, the story gives no universal answers about the meaning of life or the invaluable lessons learned from personal suffering. When faced with questions of "enlightenment" at a support group meeting, such as the stories from "other cancer survivors, the ones who write books, who speak of cancer having rearranged their priorities, bettered their relationships, made them grateful for each day," Middlebrook tries to imagine what enlightenment is, and starts to develop a list: peace, serenity, tranquility, gratitude, awe, acceptance. Then she states unequivocally, "I hate that list…I cannot exercise. I cannot make dinner. I cannot play Scrabble. I cannot read. Enlightenment is worth none of this pain."[33] Middlebrook does learn to surrender to her cancer-filled reality, but her resistance to the force of enlightenment suggests a desire to define her experience for herself, to write her own story in her own way. Unlike chaos narratives that never get better but are out of control, Middlebrook's narrative reins in the chaos and gives it a sense of order.

Third, unlike the image of the triumphant survivor who fights and wins, the author-protagonist accepts the inevitability of her death. Many diagnosed women discuss moments of lucidity when thinking about the possibility of dying before they thought they would. Several women told me about imagining their deaths, visiting their cemetery plots, planning their funerals, and writing their eulogies. Symbolic death is not the same as real death, but the experience of suffering can bring death closer to reality. Middlebrook writes: "Last year, in the transplant unit, I had decided I was going to *have* to die. I did not choose death. I just thought it was coming to me…At night, approaching sleep, I admonished myself to let go, to die if that was what happened…In the morning I was still alive."[34] Living with terminal illness, Middlebrook began to see herself not as a survivor, but as a "dier." Situating the dying process within lived experience gave her the empathy to sit with dying friends, and a sense of comfort and connection for herself: "Bless [my children, my husband, and my friends] for not turning their pain of losing me into frantic activity to keep me alive, for not abandoning me by clinging to the illusive idea of keeping me with them."

Seeing the Crab is not the typical cancer story. It is one of the discomfiting *terrible stories* saturated with realism that inhabits the fringes of pink ribbon culture. Its seemingly fragmented presentation, failure to transcend, and talk of death are taboo in pink ribbon culture. The book's capacity to bring the reader into the author's lived experience just as it is, a woman living with daily suffering from a fatal disease, reveals another pathway to survivorship that involves the practical matter of getting on with life in the face of trouble. The main character does not achieve symbolic mastery of the situation, nor is the situation frenzied or muddled. Instead, she learns how to incorporate the illness into her life. Middlebrook's communication is not meant for the masses; she speaks honestly to those who will listen.

> . . .*child, i tell you now it was not*
> *the animal blood i was hiding from,*
> *it was the poet in her, the poet and*
> *the terrible stories she could tell.*
> LUCILLE CLIFTON, "TELLING OUR STORIES"
> FROM THE TERRIBLE STORIES[35]

Throughout my discussion of realistic illness narratives, I have made reference to "the terrible stories," those ingenuous stories that are hard to tell and hard to hear, but which hold tremendous power for both the speaker and the listener to share in the gradations of challenging life experiences. The phrase refers to the title of the first book of poems that Lucille Clifton published after her breast cancer diagnosis in 1994. She opens *The Terrible Stories*[36] with the poem called "telling our stories," which directs the reader to the tone and purpose of the book: the necessity and terror of words. Clifton conveys how imagery and language have the capacity to elicit fear and understanding. Her poetry grows out of the totality of her life experiences, the obstacles she faces, her perceptions, and her understanding of evolving human conditions. Likewise, Clifton's poems about cancer reveal a personal story about who she is as a survivor.

Diagnosed at age 58 with a small malignant tumor, Clifton was told that her cancer was detected "early," and she had a lumpectomy.[37] Six years later, she had a recurrence.[38] This was not a metastasis in which the original breast cancer had spread, but a new breast cancer.[39] She had a mastectomy in 2001. In *The Terrible Stories*, Clifton portrays the life cycle of her first diagnosis. The second section of the book, "from the cadaver," is a series of nine poems, beginning with a memory of running to the telephone to hear the words "cancer...early detection...no mastectomy...not yet" ("amazons," 21), and ending with reflections on mortality ("rust" and "from the cadaver," 28-29). The poems in the middle reflect significant signposts. On the evening before surgery, there is a dream about one breast whispering softly to the other, offering solace for its impending demise ("lumpectomy eve," 22). A birthday poem titled "1994" marks the date of diagnosis, as the poet leaves her 58th year with a "cold and mortal body" and "the scar of disbelief" about "how dangerous it is to be born with breasts" (24). "Scar" accentuates the wound cancer leaves behind, what it signifies, and an awareness that the poet must learn to live with a new embodied reality (25).

Clifton's story of cancer is one of simultaneous dread, sadness, and acceptance. She illustrates the essence of breast cancer as she sees it, as both a threat to, and a veritable aspect of, her being. In "consulting the book of changes: radiation," Clifton asks a philosophical question: "what is the splendor of one breast on one woman?" (23). When she tells cancer, "you have your own story" ("1994," 24), she recognizes both its influence on her embodied experience as well as her own power to give it meaning. She mourns her wounded, irradiated body, but she does not perceive her body as an enemy to be fought. Instead, she acknowledges breast cancer's imprint even as she moves through life with it. Speaking to her scar, she writes:[40]

> we will learn
> to live together.
> i will call you
> ribbon of hunger
> and desire
> empty pocket flap
> edge of before and after.

and you

what will you call me?

. . .

Clifton conveys a realistic narrative within a poetic form, holding the middle ground between symbolism and realism. Middlebrook did the same thing using prose: "Every morning I look at the scar on my chest, where my breast used to be, every evening, every time I shower or bathe, go swimming, put on a bra, take off a bra, decide not to wear a bra. I would like not to notice, I would like not to remember, but I do."[41] Neither writer diminishes the ongoing impact of her scar, makes light of it, gets used to it, beautifies it, or transforms it to a different meaning. Their words do not conjure imagery of normalization, transcendence, or triumphant survivorship.

Within a realistic narrative, cancer is situated within the broader context of a person's life. It is a tapestry that the ill person continually re-weaves as she develops new understandings about how cancer fits within the scheme of things. Three years after *The Terrible Stories* was published, Clifton dealt with several other serious health problems.[42] She had a kidney transplant in 1997, a cancerous abdominal tumor removed in 2000, and the removal of an overactive parathyroid gland about a year later. She was diagnosed with renal cancer around the same time as her breast cancer recurrence. When she published *Mercy* in 2004, she emphasized the importance of memory in helping people to heal the wounds of life, not to rise above them but to travel with them. In addition to her new poems, Clifton recalls her earlier poems, including them as selected reprints in the collection to further expose cancer's impression on her continually evolving life. Her cancer story continued to take the past into account even as it was rewritten. Lucille Clifton died in February of 2010 at the age of 73. News stories explained that her death occurred "after a long battle with cancer."[43]

Fifteen years ago, the *New York Times Magazine* proclaimed about breast cancer that society couldn't look away anymore. Apparently, we were ready to see the damage of breast cancer. However, in that historical moment our societal gaze turned to the pink ribbon. We were not ready to see the damage or hear the terrible stories. Still, the stories continued because, as Clifton aptly wrote, "the saddest lies/are the ones we tell ourselves" ("1994," 24). Even amid the excess of triumphantly pink survivorship, realistic narratives continued to surface, image by image, journal entry by journal entry, story by story, poem by poem. While some used the resources of pink culture to communicate their stories, others did not. Without restitution, chaos, or quest, some of these authors told their own stories, in their own voices, with their own words. As they articulated their experiences, their vulnerability and authenticity gave listeners insight into aspects of survivorship that lay beneath everyday cultural scripts. They live on as a countercurrent of survivor culture, revealing yet another shade of pink.

NOTES

1. Matuschka, "Why I Did It," *Glamour Magazine*, November 1993.

2. K. Garrison, "The Personal is Rhetorical: War, Protest, and Peace in Breast Cancer Narratives," *Disability Studies Quarterly* 27, no. 4 (2007): 3.

3. Alive, Alive Oh! Performed April 17th, 2005, at Academy of Holy Names in Albany, New York, sponsored by Pen & Palette, Capital Region Action Against Breast Cancer (CRAAB!), and Theater Voices.

4. A. Frank, *The Wounded Storyteller: Body, Illness, and Ethics* (Chicago: University of Chicago, 1995).

5. M. Glaser, "I'd Like Not to Be a Stranger in the World: A Conversation/Interview with Lucille Clifton," *Antioch Review* 58, no. 3 (2000): 310-29.

6. The Breast Cancer Fund, ed., *Art.Rage.Us: Art and Writing by Women with Breast Cancer* (San Francisco: Chronicle Books, 1998).

7. New York University, "Literature, Arts, and Medicine Database: Literature Annotations" (copyright 1993-2009), http://litmed.med.nyu.edu/Annotation?action=view&annid=1515 (accessed September 28, 2009).

8. D. C. DeMille, "Circus de Vida or The Crucified Clown," http://dcdemille.home.att.net/circus_de_vida_large.htm

9. Groupstone, Inc., "Circus de Vida by Diana DeMille" (2002), http://www.inmotionmedia.net/BCAC/art/more.html (accessed September 22, 2009).

10. Groupstone, Inc., "Radiation Collage by Kit Morris" (2002), http://www.inmotionmedia.net/BCAC/art/more2.html (accessed September 22, 2009).

11. Groupstone, Inc., "Persephone's Return by Joyce Radke" (2002), http://www.inmotionmedia.net/BCAC/art/more3.html (accessed September 22, 2009).

12. Amazon.Com, "Art.Rage.Us.: Art and Writing by Women with Breast Cancer." Retrieved September 28, 2009. URL: http://www. amazon.com/Art-Rage-Us-Writing-Women-Breast-Cancer/ dp/0811821307/ref=sr_1_1?ie=UTF8&s=books&qid=1253636173&sr =1-1

13. Breast Cancer Fund, ed., "Art.Rage.Us."

14. A. Myers, *Winged Victory: Altered Images: Transcending Breast Cancer* (San Diego, CA: Photographic Gallery of Fine Art Books, 2009).

15. Jila Nikpay, *Heroines: Transformation in the Face of Breast Cancer* (New York: Zenith Services, 2006).

16. T. Lorant, *Reconstructing Aphrodite* (Syracuse, NY: Syracuse University Press, 2001).

17. Lilly USA, "Oncology on Canvas: Expressions of a Woman's Cancer Journey" (2009), http://www.lillyoncologyoncanvas.com/Pages/ Loochomepage.aspx (accessed September 29, 2009).

18. *Ibid.*

19. Lilly USA, "Lilly Oncology: Oncology on Canvas. Exhibitor's Toolkit. Oncology on Canvas Template – Media Alert" (2009), http:// www.lillyoncologyoncanvas.com/Pages/ExhibitorsToolkit.aspx (accessed September 29, 2009).

20. D. D. Coward, "Self-Transcendence and Emotional Well-Being in Women with Advanced Breast Cancer," *Oncology Nursing Forum* 18 (1991): 857-63; M. P. Mellors, J. A. Erlen, P. D. Coontz, & K. T. Lucke, "Transcending the Suffering of AIDS," *Journal of Community Health Nursing* 18, no. 4 (2001): 235-46; M. P. Mellors, T. A. Riley, & J. A. Erlen, "HIV, Self-Transcendence, and Quality of Life," *Journal of the Association of Nurses in AIDS Care* 2 (1997): 59-69; L. Ramer, D. Johnson, L. Chan, & M. T. Barrett, "The Effect of HIV/AIDS Disease Progression on Spirituality and Self-Transcendence in a Multicultural Population," *Journal of Transcultural Nursing* 17, no. 3 (2006): 280-9.

21. B. Nygren, L. Alex, E. Jonsen, Y., Gustafson, A., Norberg, & B. Lundman, "Resilience, Sense of Coherence, Purpose in Life and Self-Transcendence in Relation to Perceived Physical and Mental Health among the Oldest Old," *Aging and Mental Health* 9, no. 4 (2005): 354-62; P. G. Reed, "Toward a Nursing Theory Of Self-transcendence: Deductive Reformulation Using Developmental Theories," *Advances in Nursing Science* 13, no. 4 (1991): 64-77; M. Sanford, *Waking: A Memoir of Trauma and Transcendence* (New York: Rodale, 2006); S. Upchurch, "Self-transcendence and Activities of Daily Living: The Woman with the Pink Slippers," *Journal of Holistic Nursing* 17, no. 3 (1999): 251-66.

22. Nygren et al. "Resilience, Sense of Coherence, Purpose in Life," 355.

23. Kathy Charmaz, "'Discoveries' of Self in Illness," in *Health, Illness, and Healing: Society, Social Context, and Self,* ed. K. Charmaz & D. A. Paternati, 72-82 (Los Angeles: Roxbury, 1999); M. A. Newman, *Health as Expanding Consciousness* (2d ed.) (Boston: Jones & Bartlett, 2005).

24. Sanford, *Waking,* 5.

25. B. Ehrenreich, *Bright-sided: How the Relentless Promotion of Positive Thinking Has Undermined America* (Macmillan, 2009).

26. Lucille Clifton, *The Terrible Stories* (3rd ed.) (Rochester, NY: BOA Editions, 1994/1996).

27. Audre Lorde, *The Cancer Journals* (San Francisco: Aunt Lute Books, 1980/2006), 9.

28. *Ibid.,* 20, 23.

29. *Ibid.,* 56.

30. *Ibid.,* 74.

31. Alex De Veaux, *Warrior Poet: A Biography of Audre Lorde* (New York: W. W. Norton, 2004).

32. Christina Middlebrook, *Seeing the Crab: A Memoir of Dying* (New York: Basic Books, 1996), 203.

33. *Ibid.,* 149, 166.

34. *Ibid.*, 202.

35. Clifton, *The Terrible Stories.*

36. *Ibid.*

37. Mary Jane Lupton, *Lucille Clifton: Her Life and Letters* (New York: Praeger, 2006).

38. The standard of care is to follow the lumpectomy with 5 to 7 weeks of radiation therapy to eliminate lingering cancer cells, and women who receive this treatment are just as likely to be living 20 years after their diagnosis as women who have mastectomies.

39. Research published in the *New England Journal of Medicine* showed that 14 percent of women treated with lumpectomy plus radiation had a recurrence in the same breast. See B. Fisher, S. Anderson, J. Bryant, R. G. Margolese, M. Deutsch, E. R. Fisher, J. H. Jeong, & N. Wolmark, "Twenty-Year Follow-Up of a Randomized Trial Comparing Total Mastectomy, Lumpectomy, and Lumpectomy Plus Irradiation for the Treatment of Invasive Breast Cancer," *New England Journal of Medicine* 347, no. 6 (2002): 1233-41.

40. Clifton, *The Terrible Stories.*

41. Middlebrook, *Seeing the Crab*, 8.

42. Lupton, *Lucille Clifton.*

43. Ifill, Gwen. "Poet Lucille Clifton Dies After Cancer Battle". PBS Newshour, February 15, 2010.

NINE

RETHINKING PINK RIBBON CULTURE

It is quite possible to live with something that is broken if it is not likely to cause further damage. It may be easier and less expensive just to stick with the status quo. As individuals, we are constantly trying to discern whether our jobs, relationships, financial situations, health, lifestyles, and many other aspects of our modern lives are resulting in the quality of life we want. We assess, and sometimes agonize over, whether we will be better off in the long run if we change some aspect of our lives, or if we let it go awhile longer. Sometimes we just become accustomed to living with suboptimal situations, believing we are powerless to change them. Sometimes we resist the urge to confront problematic situations until it becomes too painfully obvious that they are working against us, damaging our very soul.

The same is true for societies. The engines of society can continue to run within institutions, organizations, and cultural systems long after their calibrations are no longer optimal, their performance has declined, and their output has become harmful. They still function on some level, but they need to be fixed to achieve optimal performance and to prevent further damage. Pink ribbon culture is one of these engines.

With good intentions, pink ribbon culture has made a promise to end breast cancer forever. Volunteers and organizations work to make this promise a reality by participating in events, raising money for research and support programs, telling their stories, speaking on behalf of breast cancer survivors, maintaining public and political interest, disseminating information, organizing support networks, shaping public policy, and conscientiously purchasing or promoting pink products and services. With so much investment and mobilization, it would seem that the pink ribbon culture were a well-oiled machine. In many ways it is, but unfortunately pink ribbon culture is also producing a set of consequences that work against its primary objective.

Pink ribbon culture has created a suboptimal situation. *Fighting the good fight* has taken precedence over winning the war. This can be hard to see because the pink ribbon has become an important and enduring symbol, a venerated icon that produces a vague but powerful "pink ribbon effect." The pink ribbon (and by extension the color pink) elicits a sequence of meanings and images that anchor a set of cherished thoughts and feelings about what it means to fight and win the war on breast cancer.

Representing all that is good about America—optimism, scientific progress, generosity, and the ability of Americans to rise to any challenge—the pink ribbon effect creates emotional allegiance to the cause of breast cancer. Emotional commitments can be more powerful and more sustaining that contractual ones.

Some of the best choices we've ever made (and perhaps some of the worst) result more from emotional responses to coincidental situations than from meticulously planned, well-evaluated proposals. Sociologist Howard Becker writes:

> Like so many people who reflect on how they met their mate, I was tremendously aware of the many things that, had they happened differently, would have sent me somewhere other than Columbia, Missouri, on the day I met [my wife.]... While everyone recognizes that stories like these are "really the way things happen"... a well-constructed story can satisfy us as an explanation.[1]

If things do "really happen" by coincidence, then why do people so often try to explain their decisions and give accounts of their behavior in rational terms?

Logic is a highly valued societal belief. Since the time of Plato and Aristotle, rationality has been more highly valued than emotion—so much so that society is organized in ways that minimize opportunities for happenstance and emotional input. Social and bureaucratic processes are designed to reduce uncertainty, and few things are considered to be less certain than relying on coincidence and emotion. Despite this deeply ingrained belief in the systems of logic, much of mental life is based on sensory-level data: a hunch, a gut feeling, an intuition. Psychologist Gerd Gigerenzer points out in the book *Gut Feelings: The Intelligence of the Unconscious*[2] that some of the most successful people rely on gut instincts to excel in their fields. Sometimes people even ignore available data and rely on gut feelings instead. Gigerenzer argues that in reality, thinking with the gut is common, even though it is rather socially unacceptable.

Maybe coincidence and intuition really are how things happen. Marketing and advertising experts think so: they spend billions of dollars developing sophisticated techniques to appeal to emotions in ways that move certain thoughts and actions to the foreground. If we think with our guts, then appealing to our guts first would be a necessary condition for marketing ideas and commodities. Yet to satisfy the societal requirement of rationality, emotional appeals would have to be coupled with some kind of information. The falsifiability of the information is not important. An ad for an expensive automobile may appeal to the desire for luxury and include an informative statement about a consumer rating. Pharmaceutical ads show fulfilling lifestyles and then include the FDA-required list of possible side effects as an informational addendum. The steady inundation of emotional appeals coupled with select informational sound bites is geared toward reinforcing core beliefs and desires. Very simply, people are more inclined to act on behalf of things they feel good about and already believe in. Using iconic symbolism, the pink ribbon effect works in similar ways.

The pink ribbon symbolizes breast cancer awareness, but it also functions as a summarizing image of a multitude of shifting meanings. In the context of pink ribbon culture, the ribbon refers to core American beliefs about optimism, scientific progress, generosity, and the ability to rise to any challenge. Once these beliefs are accessed through gut feelings (e.g., fear of breast cancer, hope for a future without breast cancer, and the good feelings that arise from fighting the good fight), a person is primed for taking some kind of conscientious action. The advertisement, public service announcement, TV show, brochure, doctor's suggestion, or even a robo-call from one's insurance carrier will suggest the action: "join the fight," "get your mammogram," "shop for the cure." To encourage people to take action, the pink ribbon draws on core beliefs to create a deep connection to the cause. However, the reality of breast cancer is difficult to grasp (i.e., unknown causes, increasing prevalence, medical uncertainty, no cure, many casualties). Likewise, the war against this mystifying enemy is equally hard to fathom and potentially too vast for anyone to imagine a clear plan of action. To close the distance between a colossal idea like the war on breast cancer and potential recruits, pink ribbon culture creates proximity to the idea. It focuses attention to the imaginary realm in which everyone envisions the ultimate end in mind, a future without breast cancer.

The vision of future victory in the war against breast cancer is reiterated throughout pink ribbon culture in slogans such as "End breast cancer forever;" "Imagine life without breast cancer;"

"Let's make breast cancer obsolete;" "Erase it for good." Since potential recruits are not in a position to know for themselves how this laudable victory will be achieved, pink ribbon culture helps us to establish proximal relationships with the people who are.[3] The experts in the war on breast cancer are those who have been touched by breast cancer (survivors and their loved ones) and those with medical authority.

As the generic breast cancer survivor, the she-ro provides access to the vision. The she-ro of today approximates the victory of tomorrow. An American Airlines press release about its partnership with Komen for the Cure includes a symbolically significant statement similar to almost every write-up on the foundation I have seen. It brings forth pink ribbon culture's vision through the she-roic promise of a sister:

> Nancy G. Brinker promised her dying sister, Susan G. Komen, that she would do everything in her power to end breast cancer forever. In 1982, that promise became Susan G. Komen for the Cure® and launched the global breast cancer movement.[4]

Susan Komen's biography, as Brinker tells it on the Komen website, recounts Suzy's courageous struggle with breast cancer, upholding all of the elements of the she-ro, including optimism, good humor, and conventional treatment. Numerous descriptions of the foundation emphasize Brinker's promise to her dying sister. Using the present tense (dying) brings Susan Komen's life into the frame. The promise occurred while her sister was still alive, still a survivor. This distinction is vital as it

extracts the she-ro's vision while simultaneously calling attention to the reality of Komen's impending death. The worst
thing a person can ask about any war is whether those who died,
died in vain. If they did, then the war was not worth fighting.
Memorializing those who have died from breast cancer awakens
the urgency and importance of the war. We grieve with Brinker
about the loss of her sister and relate to making promises to
those we love, thereby increasing the chances that we will
develop an emotive allegiance to the cause itself.

We also gain access to the vision through a proximal relationship with medical authorities and the medical system as a
whole. Every day there are new reports about better advances
that lead to new medical breakthroughs. *Forbes.com* recently
reported "a revolution brewing in pharmacology…We are
beginning to understand why certain drugs work better, worse
or not at all for certain patients. This breakthrough is being
made possible by the wealth of new genomic data that is generated every day."[5] In the context of the vision, we are to assume
that incremental progress will ultimately end in "cures." Victory
achieved. Supporting the vision reinforces the core belief that
scientific progress will prevail, leading to optimism and pride in
American ingenuity. Amid scores of similar messages that share
this sentiment, we are more likely to listen when a person with
medical expertise tells us that one day mothers will no longer
have to worry about their daughters getting breast cancer. We
want to believe. Most importantly, there is no way to disprove
the statement, so it continues to support the vision.

Proximal relationships enable people to embrace the vision of ending breast cancer forever without having to know realistically how this will happen. By relying on the vision and the senses, the pink ribbon effect eludes empirical justification. When information is provided, it serves as an appendage used to support the vision rather than a roadmap that will achieve the goal. All we need to know is that we can rely on Nancy Brinker to keep her promise to her sister and on cutting-edge science to find the cures.

With pink ribbon culture operating so well on the symbolic level, it does not need to establish validity or provide falsifiable evidence. Although the medical enterprise itself is based on a commitment to rational discourse and evidence-based conclusions, this is not its primary function in pink ribbon culture. Information is used to corroborate sensory responses and reinforce existing beliefs to create the pink ribbon effect. Those who reach different conclusions, even with scientific evidence, are a threat to the culture. In the same article in *The New York Times* that addressed the American Cancer Society's eventual acknowledgment that it had exaggerated the benefits of mammography screening, Dr. Peter Albertsen of the University of Connecticut Health Center explained why it would be so difficult to make such statements. He said, "If you question overdiagnosis in breast cancer, you are against women." Albertsen's candid statement reveals an outcome of the pink ribbon effect: opposing those who provide access to the vision fuels another kind of war, an *us/them* scenario in which friends of the cause are pitted against enemies of the cause. If you're not with us, you're against us.

The pink ribbon effect has made it so that the pink ribbon *culture* is generally beyond critique. The hot issue of the day is whether corporate cause-marketing raises money for the cause, *not* whether the cause (as it is currently structured) is actually achieving its goals, or whether the culture itself is producing detrimental effects that go beyond companies and major organizations increasing their revenues while dropping dollars into a pink trough. Cause-marketing does raise money, and some of it goes toward research studies and support/education programs, but seldom do we see any details about where the money flows and the results it allegedly generates. Dr. Larry Norton of Memorial-Sloan Kettering Cancer Center assures the readers of *Delta Sky Magazine*[6] that "there's a direct line between all those pink products and money that [he's] seeing used for extraordinary high-quality research." When asked to extract exactly how much of the approximately $6 billion raised from industry and the philanthropic community actually goes to breast cancer research, he says that "the lines are just too amorphous and fuzzy" because "science simply doesn't work that way." Dr. Norton can make such contradictory statements because as the medical director of the Evelyn H. Lauder Breast Cancer at Sloan, he *is* that direct line between industry and research. This vantage point gives the reader access to the vision while reinforcing, once again, the pink ribbon effect.

Pink consumers are supposed to feel good about consumptive virtue, not ask inconvenient questions about how, when, where, or to what end all of the money is used. Nor should consumers ask whether society is getting any closer to achieving the pink ribbon culture's vision of a world without breast cancer. The pink ribbon effect assures everyone that we can trust the leaders of pink ribbon culture to know what they are doing.

In and of itself, there is nothing inherently wrong with pink passion or conscientious consumption. The pink ribbon culture has used these strategies to garner extensive funding, recognition, and power. But if the eradication of breast cancer is the goal, we need to know about the consequences (intended and unintended) of pink ribbon culture's, and hence society's, mechanisms for dealing with breast cancer, and work toward minimizing the damages and building on the successes. The countercurrents of pink ribbon culture have been doing this since the beginnings of the culture's ascendancy. Cultural resistance and formal organizing have existed alongside pink ribbon culture, sometimes using the culture's resources for their own purposes and sometimes working in direct opposition. Looking to these efforts will help to light a new path toward a future without breast cancer.

"NOT JUST RIBBONS"

In 2002, the National Breast Cancer Coalition (NBCC) created the "Not Just Ribbons" national campaign to move attention away from simple "awareness" messages and toward substantive policy issues such as genetic discrimination, access to cancer therapies, breast cancer and the environment, and a meaningful patient bill of rights. A series of advertisements printed in national magazines did not include ribbons but instead showed a bulldozer, toolbox, and hardhat to make the point that the symbols used in breast cancer advocacy needed to align with a broader message that the war on breast cancer required concerted political action. In the fall 2002 newsletter that launched the campaign, NBCC President Fran Visco explained that her remarks about ribbons were often misconstrued. She said, "Not for one moment would I ask our members to throw away their ribbons. My concern is focused on those who simply wear one—without the concurrent commitment to do the 'heavy lifting'.[7] I believe they are deluding themselves if they believe a symbol is all it takes to eradicate this disease." A national poll commissioned by the NBCC found that indeed support for the cause and the ribbon was substantial, but the symbolic support did not necessarily carry with it a commitment to political action. The winter newsletter reported that "while 96 percent of Americans agree that breast cancer is a critical health problem and 50 percent believe that wearing a pink ribbon is an effective tool to fight breast cancer, only six percent have contacted their elected officials on issues concerning breast cancer."[8]

The "Not Just Ribbons" campaign aligned with NBCC's belief that the eradication of breast cancer would be possible only with increased environmental research and intervention, improvements in access to cancer therapies, and nondiscrimination in insurance. The legislative agenda the coalition put forth supported these beliefs. The coalition also called for a patient bill of rights that included coverage for routine healthcare costs associated with clinical trials, access to the right providers, involvement in treatment decisions based on good science, confidentiality of their health information, and the right to receive accurate information about their health plans. While the NBCC's publicity against the pink ribbon did not continue, the legislative agenda did, along with consumer advocacy training and public outreach to provide patient-centered and evidence-based analyses of breast cancer research and controversies.

The NBCC has been in the forefront of providing analyses, position papers, and fact sheets about scientific research and health delivery practices. With the goal of eradication in mind, the coalition prioritizes the use of scientific evidence to measure progress. Similar to many of the environmentally focused breast cancer organizations, NBCC advocates collaboration with the scientific community on the development and implementation of new research models and clinical trials. NBCC's Project LEAD, for example, is a short course that teaches laypersons to understand biomedical technoscience in ways that enable them to make informed decisions and participate in peer-review boards that fund breast cancer research. NBCC focuses on the vision of eradication just as the pink ribbon culture does. The difference is that instead of using medical authority as an addendum to corroborate feelings of commitment to the cause, NBCC, along with the environmental breast cancer movement, evaluates scientific evidence and uses it to develop critical analyses and collective actions.

"THINK BEFORE YOU PINK"

Breast Cancer Action (BCA) in the San Francisco Bay area was one of the first organizations to raise awareness about the cancer industry and continues to be in the forefront of efforts to reveal the conflict of interest between industries that raise money for breast cancer while also profiting from breast cancer, contributing to carcinogenic environmental conditions, and/or weakening environmental and occupational regulations that may decrease cancer incidence. The organization implicated the American Cancer Society in a 1990 newsletter with a report that highlighted several controversies surrounding the society's approach to breast cancer. These included the refusal to take a stand against environmental carcinogens, ties to the treatment-oriented medical profession (including that the society held a portion of the patent for a frequently used chemotherapy agent, 5-fluorouracil), attempts to discourage research, and efforts to mislead the public with statistics alternatively used to generate fear and hope.[9] They even included a review of Ralph Moss's *The Cancer Industry*, providing more evidence of concern about conventional approaches to treatment.[10] Nearly 20 years later, the American Cancer Society has just started to acknowledge environmental links to cancer and only recently admitted to exaggerated promises about the benefits of mammography screening.

BCA condemned the industry again in 1995, this time with a focus on National Breast Cancer Awareness Month (NBCAM).

As a key sponsor of NBCAM, the American Cancer Society was implicated once again for its ties to industry. The article also cited Zeneca's sponsorship of the program. As a manufacturer of the hormone therapy drug tamoxifen and a major producer of chlorine and petroleum-based products, BCA questioned Zeneca's influence on NBCAM's promotional materials, suggesting that corporate interests may account for the fact that the word "carcinogen" does not even appear in any of NBCAM's information. BCA reiterated this information repeatedly in newsletters and other information sources and now gets the point across by referring to NBCAM as National Breast Cancer *Industry* Month—a slick public relations campaign that avoids discussion of the causes and prevention of breast cancer and instead focuses on "awareness" as a way to encourage women to get their mammograms.

BCA's exposé of the industry highlighted not only corporate profits from breast cancer but also the role of corporations in contributing to environmental conditions that produce breast cancer and other cancers in the first place. The organization coined the term "pinkwashing" to describe companies that raise funds for breast cancer while diverting attention from the company's potential hazards, such as producing chemicals or toxins that have been linked to the disease. Charging these companies with pinkwashing, however, also implicates the breast cancer organizations that are willing to accept donations and form partnerships with them. Although BCA refuses to accept corporate contributions from pharmaceutical companies, chemical manufacturers, oil companies, tobacco companies, health insurance agencies, cancer treatment facilities, or corporate entities whose products or manufacturing processes directly endanger environmental and/or occupational health or may possibly contribute to cancer incidence, many other organizations (especially in pink ribbon culture) do not make this distinction.[11] Economic constraints have encouraged pinkwashing and large organizations in pink ribbon culture use it to fuel the pink machine.

BCA's "Think Before You Pink" campaign called for transparency and accountability on the part of companies that take part in breast cancer fundraising and encouraged consumers to ask critical questions about pink ribbon promotions. With the large and growing number of individuals and companies aligning with the breast cancer cause, it is nearly impossible to tell how much money is being spent on breast cancer research and whether those funds are being well spent. The fuzzy line just keeps getting fuzzier. But that's not all: the money that is raised through pink cause-marketing is primarily going to huge foundations that are already wealthy, may have questionable ties with the cancer industry and corporate polluters, and tend to ignore or trivialize the preponderance of scientific evidence that calls for significant changes in society's approach to breast cancer. As the environmental movements have discovered, funneling funds entirely into screening programs and cure research will not move society any closer to eliminating the causes of breast cancer.

Using pink ribbon symbolism against itself, the "Think Before You Pink" campaign also draws attention to the use of pink stereotyping to sell products. Gemma Tarlach writes: "And nowhere, perhaps aside from Hooters, is that equation more ingrained than in the breast cancer industry, a monolith marketed by corporate America that reinforces stereotypes about what it means to be a woman. Woman = breast = pink."[12] Pink cause-marketing is rife with examples. The year 2009 marks the 8th Annual Blogger Boobie-Thon in which bloggers from around the world send in photos of their breasts (covered and uncovered) to help raise money for breast cancer research.[13] T-shirts read: "I love breasts;" "Stop the war in my-rack;" and "Save the tatas." Men's versions of the T-shirts (complete with a pink ribbon) read: "Tatas are awesome" and "If loving tatas is wrong, I don't wanna be right."[14] Pin-up calendars of nude "co-eds" to raise money for the cause are not a far cry from Ford's Warrior campaign that features young, busty she-ros in pink.

The cultural equation of breasts, and having breasts, with women's heterosexual identity enables pink ribbon products to trivialize and ignore the realities of breast cancer while simultaneously degrading women and putting them in their place. As a form of resistance, the Breast Cancer Fund's "Obsessed with Breasts" campaign created a series of shocking advertisements meant to challenge the objectification of the female breast. The campaign took famous ads by Victoria's Secret, Cosmopolitan magazine, and Obsession perfume and superimposed photographs of mastectomy scars on the models. The Breast Cancer Fund argued that "until the culture more appropriately honors women and their bodies, we will never defeat a disease that attacks its most profound symbol of sexuality and nurture."[15] Reminiscent of Matuschka's "Beauty Out of Damage" photograph, the campaign was designed to provoke the public toward greater involvement in issues that tend to be overlooked in pink ribbon culture.

Sexualizing women in the name of breast cancer is only one of the detrimental consequences of many pink ribbon campaigns. They also infantilize women and emphasize their traditional social roles. Teddy bears, rubber duckies, and M&Ms are used to comfort and pacify children, yet companies sell them to grown women in the name of the cause. A portion of the sales of Pink Ribbon Barbie Doll by Mattel will benefit the Susan G. Komen Breast Cancer Foundation. Wearing a pink gown with a signature pink ribbon pinned to her shoulder, Pink Ribbon Barbie is supposed to be a tool to help those affected with breast cancer talk to girls and a way to support the cause.[16] Barbara Ehrenreich pointed out many years ago that it would be unconscionable to give Matchbox cars to men with prostate cancer.[17] It's as if femininity is incompatible with adulthood, unless of course the adult women are in their proper place, cooking, cleaning, and satisfying the needs of others with pink kitchen aids, pink vacuum cleaners, pink cosmetics, and other feminine accessories.

These kinds of pink products and symbols reinforce the notion that breast cancer is a danger only because it threatens women's sexual identity and men's access to their breasts, and the pink ribbon effect generally guarantees a pink ribbon seal of approval. Traditional femininity has already been integrated into pink ribbon culture, casting women's empowerment in terms of lipstick choices, shoes, and pink buckets of chicken. Fundraising has become the only priority. And the mandate for optimism enables women's subjugation to be cast under the umbrella of humor. The credo that laughter is the best medicine is easier to accommodate than, as Audre Lorde said 30 years ago, "real food and clean air and a saner future on a liveable earth!"[18] Pink ribbon symbolism not only distracts the public from the harsh realities of breast cancer and the actions that would be necessary to move toward its eradication, it also produces a feel-good culture in which the idea that breast cancer is a good cause translates to a belief that supporting it is a good thing that will always lead to good outcomes. The pink ribbon effect demonizes and isolates those who do not happily accept all of the pink goodness the culture has to offer.

One of the most compelling illustrations of this dimension of the pink ribbon effect is the story of Paula at one of the National Race for the Cure events. Paula was diagnosed with an invasive breast cancer and had three recurrences. She was in stage 4 of the disease when I met her, and the cancer had moved to her lungs. We met through a mutual acquaintance, and Paula knew I was writing a book about pink ribbon culture. She was very interested about what I had learned so far, and she wanted to make sure that I knew her take on it. She said, "You know, it's not what it's cracked up to be." I asked her to explain, and she told me the story of the last time she ever went to public fundraising event for breast cancer.

> I went to the National Race for the Cure….Everyone was excit-
> ed…Survivors had to wear…pink hats, so I wore mine. People
> were writing…the names of people they knew with breast can-
> cer, or people they had lost [on their t-shirts]…I looked up and
> saw my name…I went up to [this woman] to ask…why my
> name was on her t-shirt…She said, "well they told us write the
> name of a survivor…I didn't know anyone, but I saw your name
> on someone else's shirt, so I wrote it on mine too." She smiled.
> I didn't. I said, "But, you don't even know me." She smiled again
> and replied, "Well, I want to support you anyway." I walked
> away…feeling like a tool. She didn't know me… But, she was
> going to use my name to make her feel good about supporting
> this cause. I left, and never went to a race again.

Paula's experience captures one of the most personally dev-astating sides of pink ribbon organizing. The generic survivor has become so central to pink ribbon culture that any survivor will do. A name on a T-shirt or a pink hat is all we need to hap-pily fight the war on breast cancer. The personal struggle of the disease is left on the sidelines, transformed to a transcendent story, or left back at home where no one will ever see.

Paula told me more about the tyranny of pink ribbon cul-ture, how it usurped the voices of so many diagnosed women. She tried to keep her story her own. She even sent a periodic newsletter to a select group of people in her inner circle because she "felt better about being able to express [her] news herself rather than rely on others, who with the best of intentions might miss a key point in the medical update or filter [her] condition through their lens." Paula's careful method of communication was an efficient attempt to guard against the misunderstandings and misinterpretations possible in any form of communication, to keep her personal business personal. It was a way to keep others from appropriating her story. In pink ribbon culture, the personal may no longer be political, but it is definitely public. Silence about breast cancer has been replaced with full disclosure (using the proper filters and accepted storyline).

If we ask whether the "ends" justify the "means" in how pink ribbon culture has approached breast cancer, we must look at all of the "ends" before making that determination. Is it enough to raise a lot of money if it enables corporations to keep polluting the environment and selling products and technologies that create profits but do not sufficiently decrease incidence and mortality? If it enables large foundations to claim the voice of the breast cancer movement without being responsive to the multitude of truly grassroots organizations who are caring for their local communities and organizing for real social change? If it limits how we think and talk about breast cancer and dis-authenticates the diversity of experiences that inhabit survivorship?

If it exploits pink femininity to disempower, demean, and objectify women? If it uses she-roism to enforce optimism and medical compliance to practices that lead to overdiagnosis and overtreatment? If it uses fear-mongering to generate hope and a pink lifestyle that is more highly valued than the lives of those diagnosed with breast cancer? If it has not resulted in the primary objective of eradication of the disease? If it memorializes those who have died to justify a never-ending war?

The conventional wisdom in pink ribbon culture is to keep going as we've been going, and to spread the message of the pink ribbon around the globe. As breast cancer incidence rates continue to rise steadily in developing and developed countries, public health programs struggle to determine how best to deal with the growing cancer burden. Given that known risk factors only account for a small percentage of total breast cancer cases, the World Health Organization recognizes that focusing prevention strategies only on modifiable health behaviors is a limitation. Similarly, the WHO acknowledges that the widespread mammography screening of populations is not likely to reduce overall mortality. Yet the pink mainstream remains committed to a version of awareness that centers on early detection through population screening and pink ribbon community building. Taking a road less pink requires fundamental changes in the way we organize around breast cancer and in the questions we are willing to ask of ourselves, our families, our elected officials, our corporations, our medical system, our scientists, our media, and those who represent us in advocacy. If we take this road it will, I believe, make a difference.

NOTES

1. H. Becker, *Tricks of the Trade: How to Think about Your Research While You're Doing It* (Chicago: University of Chicago Press, 1998), 31.

2. G. Gigerenzer, *Gut Feelings: The Intelligence of the Unconscious* (New York: Penguin Books, 2007), 1.

3. The discussion of iconic symbolism to produce proximal relationships to an uncertain vision builds on K. Ferguson's October 20, 2009 presentation to the Texas Woman's University Women's Studies Department, "Bush in Drag: Sarah Palin and Endless War."

4. Business Wire, "American Airlines/Susan G. Komen for the Cure® Promise Grant to the University of Texas M. D. Anderson Cancer Center Enables Much Progress in First Year." http://www.businesswire.com/portal/site/home/permalink/?ndmViewId=news_view&newsId=20091015005742&newsLang=en (accessed October 15, 2009).

5. J. Turner, "The Best Medications For Your Genes." *Forbes.com,* October 27, 2009. http://www.forbes.com/2009/10/27/pharmacology-genes-medications-technology-breakthroughs-oreilly.html.

6. M. Frazier, "When did Consumption Become a Virtue? Pink," *deltaskymag.com* (October 2009), 59-65.

7. National Breast Cancer Coalition. *Call to Action* Fall (2002). http://www.stopbreastcancer.org/index.php?option=com_content&task=view&id=646.

8. National Breast Cancer Coalition. *Call to Action* Winter (2002). http://www.stopbreastcancer.org/index.php?option=com_content&task=view&id=646.

9. Breast Cancer Action, "Report: American Cancer Society." *Breast Cancer Action Newsletter* #2 October (1990), http://bcaction.org/index.php?page=newsletter-2e.

10. Breast Cancer Action, "Books to Read," *Breast Cancer Action Newsletter* #2 October (1990) http://bcaction.org/index.php?page=newsletter-2c.

11. Breast Cancer Action, "Policy on Corporate Contributions," http://bcaction.org/index.php?page=policy-on-corporate-contributions (accessed October 31, 2009).

12. G. Tarlach, "Seeing Red When Told to Think-Pink." *Breast Cancer Action Newsletter* #76 March/April (2003), 3.

13. Boobie-Thon 2001-2009, "We Share Because We Care." http://www.boobiethon.com/about/ (accessed October 30, 2009).

14. http://www.savethetatas.com/graphicpages/this_guy.html (accessed October 30, 2009).

15. The Breast Cancer Fund, Press Statement, "'Obsessed with Breasts' Ad Campaign" (2000) http://www.breastcancerfund.org/site/c.kwKXLdPaE/b.84636/k.1BD1/Press_Statement_about_the_Obsessed_with_Breasts_Campaign.htm.

16. Amazon.com 1996-2009, "Mattel Pink Ribbon Barbie," http://www.amazon.com/Barbie-Collector-Pink-Ribbon-Doll/dp/B000ERVLV6 (Accessed October 31, 2009); R. Traister, "Breast Cancer Barbie: October Brings Barbie and Breast Cancer Awareness," *Salon.com* (2006). http://www.salon.com/mwt/broadsheet/2006/10/03/breast_cancer_barbie/ (Accessed October 31, 2009).

17. B. Ehrenreich, "Welcome to Cancerland," *Harper's Magazine* (2001).

18. A. Lorde, *The Cancer Journals*, 74.

INDEX